It's a Miracle, I'm Still Sick: Growing in Faith When You Don't Get Healed

By Rev. Dan Gottwerth

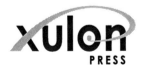

Acknowledgments

"Let me say first that I thank my God through Jesus Christ for all of you..." Romans 1:8

➤ I originally asked Eileen Evans, who was one of Lori's closest friends, to be the editor of this project. It wasn't long before we both realized that it would need more than editing. Eileen interviewed me, reworked large sections of the book, and created all the material for the Bible study. I am grateful beyond words for her partnering with me in the creation of this work and for her countless hours of rewrites. "...your Father who sees what is done in secret will reward you" (Matthew 6:6). Thank you so much for your labor of love in Lori's honor.

➤ To Matt Steinruck and Lynn Staton for making the book cover something to remember. And to Debbie Falcone for her beautiful photography of our family. They are priceless! Thank you friends.

➢ To Pastor Jon Swenson who was my mentor, friend and the voice of God to me when Heaven was silent. He not only stood beside me through the most painful time of my life, he publicly and prophetically challenged me at Lori's funeral to "write the book". How did you know?

➢ To my beautiful wife, Deb, who constantly amazed me with her unwavering support and unconditional love throughout this project. I am so in love with you! Thank you for desiring God's best for my life. "She is clothed with strength and dignity...when she speaks, her words are wise" (Proverbs 31:25-26).

➢ To our Lord and Savior Jesus Christ who wept with us and understood our grief. Thank you God for making it clear that this was *your* plan for me at this season of my life. Your timing is always perfect!

Contents

Eight
Unconditional Love......64

Nine
Welcome Home......69

Ten
Looking Forward......77

Bible Study......91

A note from the author

Welcome. The journey you are about to take will lead you through a love story. You will have a very personal view of Lori and me as we walk together through the greatest joys and the deepest sorrows life can bring. You will also get to look deeply into another love story, the love that God has for each of us. His guiding hand and protective embrace are always close to us. It is my prayer that by the end of this book you will have a deeper realization that you too are in a love story with the living God.

The format of this book is a unique combination of a story coupled with a bible study/pastoral reflection. It is my intent to give you a chance to hear from God because He wants to speak to you in your unique circumstance. The story is meant to inspire you to put your faith in a God who does not abandon you. The study portion is meant to strengthen you for your own journey. The story, along with the study, will provide you with a greater understanding of how much God loves you and how much He wants to be involved in the deepest matters of your heart.

Dan Gottwerth
www.dangottwerth.com

1

One Plus One Equals One

Two are better than one...
Ecclesiastes 4:9

The beauty of the sun setting on the western horizon always makes for a peaceful ending to a day. It's even better when you're young, full of energy and travelling west on a motorcycle to be with the woman you love. This horizon was one I couldn't wait to get to. Lori and I were both in college, but at two different schools. My school was in a fast paced, growing suburban town and hers was in a simple rural setting. The two were only 60 miles apart. It took about an hour to get there by car. An hour isn't normally that long of a drive, but to me it was too long and too far to be away. I couldn't wait to get there on the weekends to spend every minute with the beautiful woman who had captured my heart. Lori was everything I had ever dreamed of. She loved God, was beautiful, well spoken and always took the time to look nice whether "hanging around" or going out. She tirelessly dedicated herself to help others mature personally and spiritually. She was committed to hard work and had firm control over her life.

We were in college and didn't have too much money so we spent a lot of time talking over dorm-room Mac-n-cheese dinners. We took long walks late into the night around campus sharing the funny and serious stories of life. On occasion we even played miniature golf. During our first miniature golf game I had taken a significant lead but on the 12th hole, she took matters into her own hands. Her first shot landed the ball right into the middle of a small shallow creek. She was not willing to lose a stroke so she just marched straight into that creek in her nice sneakers and took her shot. I couldn't believe it! But that was Lori. When she made up her mind, there was no standing in her way.

This was an important time for our relationship as we grew together without the pressures that come with serious dating. After about a year of really getting to know each other it became clear that we wanted to take our friendship to a new level. We started dating with the idea that the friendship we had forged might turn into marriage. I had promised her that we would date no more than a year and at that time I believed that God would show us whether we had a relationship that was meant to last a lifetime.

More important conversations came up at this time like finances, children, career options, where we might want to live and what kind of lifestyle we anticipated. We took advantage of activities around campus like Inter-Varsity Christian Fellowship, concerts, picnicking along the bank of the campus pond or grabbing a quick burger at the student center. We learned valuable lessons during these early days about depending on God as the sole provider.

As time passed our love for each other grew. There was a night when Lori was studying for finals and I could tell by the sound of her voice that she was under a great deal of stress. I picked up three roses and carefully hid them inside my jacket. I presented them to her along with a neck and upper back massage. She brought up that experience often as being one of the turning points in our relationship. Lori said that it was in the small things that love was best communicated. Our love for each other grew so strong that we were sure it would last a lifetime.

I went to jeweler's row in the city and carefully picked out a ring and made reservations at an elegant and romantic French restaurant. The night was perfect and is forever etched on my heart. I'm sure the horizon was shining brighter than ever, as I was drove to Lori's school to take her to dinner. I wrote this poem for her along the way:

The time has come the day is here
When God erases all our fear
I with you, you with me, united together eternally
For on this night I commit to you
My selfless love, so simple but true;
And so one flesh we shall be
If you, Lori, will marry me.

She said yes and we started making plans for the wedding. We took our time planning and enjoyed every minute of the season we were in. During that time, we prayed a lot and sang together. We attended plays, went out to dinner and the movies. Some of the best times were spent at Longwood Gardens, which has 1,000 acres of gardens, woodlands and meadows. We enjoyed long, romantic walks through the grounds, the beautiful fountains and reading our favorite books together. One of the earliest collections that we read together was the work of James Herriot, which detailed the story of an English veterinarian who took his practice on the road through the English countryside. The book titles came from each line of an old hymn:

All things bright and beautiful,
All creatures great and small,
All things wise and wonderful:
The Lord God made them all.

We loved to read books that are in a series. We enjoyed authors like Celtic fictional writer Stephen Lawhead and suspense thriller writer Frank Peretti. When we weren't at Longwood Gardens we could be found teaching Junior High Sunday school or acting as chaperones for various youth events. We felt the closest when we served together. The year of our engagement was a year of joy, love and anticipation of what was ahead. Lori spent time shopping for the perfect dress and tasting cake. I spent time helping her do whatever she needed done.

Finally the time drew near and we began the final preparations before the ceremony. We carefully chose a verse for the program.

Two are better than one because they have a good
    return for their work:
If one falls down, his friend can help him up.
But pity the man who falls and has no one to help
    him up!
Also, if two lie down together, they will keep warm.
But how can one keep warm alone?
Though one may be overpowered, two can defend
    themselves.
A cord of three strands is not quickly broken.
(Ecclesiastes 4:9-12)

God was the third strand included in our union and this
verse seemed to reflect our intent for the day.

The big moment finally arrived. I was very nervous
as I took my place at the front of the church and waited.
The music started and the congregation waited impa-
tiently. The bride's maids made their way down the
aisle and it seemed like an eternity. Finally, the doors
were opened and Lori appeared in the entranceway.
She literally took my breath away as she glided down
the aisle. She was beautiful from every angle. I have
to admit I even choked back a tear when I saw her.
Her father kissed her and put her hand in mine and
we stepped up toward the pastor. He started the ceremony but I just couldn't take my eyes off of Lori. We
held hands tightly and tried to focus on what was
being said. We committed ourselves to each other and
to God for better or for worse, for richer or poorer in
sickness and in health 'til death do us part. Amen and
let the party begin.

With the wedding day behind us we stole away
together for a honeymoon to remember. We were on

top of the world. We had all the goodness of life ahead of us. When we returned home we settled into life together working, saving and planning our future. After three years of building a strong marital foundation we made the announcement all potential grandparents want to hear, Lori was pregnant with our first child. Rachel was born and she added even more love to the family, if that were even possible. I was determined to make sure that my relationship with Lori was stronger than ever. I really felt the pressure that comes with the responsibility of a baby, so I recommitted myself to being the best husband and father possible. I guarded my new family very carefully so Rachel could grow to be emotionally, spiritually and physically healthy. Lori was very happy and committed herself wholeheartedly to this very difficult, yet rewarding job. Taking care of a new baby was a ton of work, but she made the necessary adjustments and sacrifices all first time moms make. We embraced our new role as a team and all seemed to be well with our world.

Soon after Rachel was born we found out she was pregnant again. Lori wasn't really sure she was ready to take on the responsibility of a second child. We firmly believed, though, that God would give us the grace we needed to provide for another little life. He had other plans though. Not long into the pregnancy and for reasons we are unsure of we lost the baby. Lori was overwhelmed with grief and it took a lot of talking to work through the loss. God's grace was sufficient for us we just didn't expect it to be through these circumstances.

Three years later God blessed us again with another baby. Joshua was born in 1993. He added more love and joy to the family and our house was full and overflowing.

We were abundantly blessed and thankful for all that God had done for us. The Bible tells us that children are a gift from God and they certainly were. We felt sure that this was the right number of children for us.

Not long after Josh's birth, I revealed to Lori a desire that had been growing in my heart; I wanted to go to seminary. I had been thinking for a long time that I might go, and felt sure this was the direction God was leading me. After a lot of prayer and discussion I decided to enroll in classes. Around the same time I took a job at a local church as children's pastor. Going to school and switching jobs was a big step for us since we already had a lot on our plate. It was the right decision, though, and life moved along very busily yet peacefully and seemed to be going just as we dreamed it would. The kids were growing, our marriage was strong and we were hopeful about the future. Life went on for several years with nothing more eventful than the usual bumps in the road life may bring. All of this was about to change.

2

Those Aren't Bats in the Belfry

"Day after day and night after night they keep on saying, "Holy, holy, holy is the Lord God, the Almighty—the one who always was, who is, and who is still to come."
Revelation 4:7-8

It was a warm and beautiful, Sunday morning on a bright summer day. The family and I got up as we always did and made our way through the challenges of getting ready for church. With a heroic victory behind us we headed out for Bethlehem United Methodist Church. I was serving as the children's pastor full time and leading worship once a month. We arrived an hour early giving me time to focus and prepare to lead worship at 9 am. Rachel and Josh headed off to Sunday school and Lori along with the other members of the worship team took the stage. Lori had a beautiful alto voice and the ability to pick out harmony to just about any song. Not to mention her serious tambourine playing, which was a big help to me in keeping a steady tempo. I needed her in so many ways.

"The miracle at Bethlehem United Methodist Church" as I call it, is a day I'll never forget. As we were coming to the end of one of the songs I noticed Lori's voice dropping out. I passed it off as a monitor or mic problem and continued singing,

"We are moment, you are forever, Lord of the Ages, God before time. We are a vapor, You are eternal love everlasting, reigning on high. Holy, holy Lord God Almighty. Worthy is..."

In the middle of the chorus, Lori's voice went completely silent. Even one of her friends in the congregation noticed and commented later that she had tears streaming down her face as she gazed at the rafters. Her friend said, "I could see she was totally consumed with the experience, completely surrendered and wrapped in God's presence." I had to wait until the end of worship to find out what went wrong. As it turned out nothing was wrong at all, something good had happened. After the closing prayer, Lori and I slipped down into the first pew and I leaned over and quietly asked her what happened. "I saw angels" was her only explanation. I sat there stunned. I never expected to hear that. "Angels? You've got to be kidding", I thought. Lori was not one that focused on supernatural experiences. She graduated from college with a Latin degree magna cum laude. She was a no-nonsense lady, a very concrete thinker. Seeing angels just wasn't her style. "Angels? Where?" I asked. "Up there, in the rafters" as she pointed overhead to the area where the 150 year old wood beams were exposed. "I couldn't make out their faces, but I could tell they were singing as well as dancing in a circle." I never doubted what she saw, but have to admit I was a little disappointed that I didn't get to share that with her. I knew from Scripture that God never revealed angels to people without a purpose. For Stephen, he needed the vision of Heaven in order to sustain him during a fatal stoning in Acts 7. Lori saw angels when we were singing a song taken directly out of Revelation. The angels before God's throne regularly sing the same words from our song. This was revealed in John's vision.

> "Then I looked and heard the voice of many angels, numbering thousands upon thousands, and ten thousand times ten thousand. They encircled the throne and the living creatures and the elders. In a loud voice they sang: "Worthy is the Lamb, who was slain, to receive power and wealth and wisdom and strength and honor and glory and praise!" Revelation 5:11-12

> "Each of the four living creatures had six wings and was covered with eyes all around, even under his wings. Day and night they never stop staying: "Holy, holy, holy is the Lord God Almighty, who was, and is, and is to come Revelation 4:7-8 NIV

I knew that day something very special was happening and God was very close to us.

The lazy days of summer drifted to an end and Labor Day marked the unofficial decline of summer fun. We celebrated at a picnic with my sister and her family in the Poconos Mountains north of Philadelphia. It was a great day filled with the usual holiday fun. Toward the end of the visit, Lori was stepping out of the house and missed a small step. She twisted her ankle. We immediately elevated and iced it. She was embarrassed by the attention. She was more accustomed to doing for others but she graciously received the help. Later we got her into the car to go home. It was toward the end of the day and the shadows fell long on the road home.

She spent the next few days resting. On the morning of September 11, like so many others in the country, we turned on the TV to discover that terrorists had attacked Washington and New York. We were glued to the television as the Twin Towers came down, passenger heroes brought down flight 93 in a Pennsylvania field and the Pentagon was attacked. We were totally caught up in this national tragedy and participated in the prayer services and community gatherings that took place afterward. Lori continued to hobble to the different events that were taking place, but we never noticed that her ankle really wasn't getting any stronger. When the shock started to wane and people refocused on daily activities we realized that she needed to contact a doctor.

3

Unanswered Questions

" He personally carried our sins in His body on the cross so that we can be dead to sin and live for what is right. By His wounds you are healed."

1 Peter 2:24

Autumn brought with it the usual routine as well as a variety of changes and challenges. I had my pastoral duties and graduate classes. Lori had a full-time administrative position in a counseling office. The kids were in school and had their activities. Lori went to see the doctor again to try to determine why her ankle wasn't any stronger. He scheduled her for regular physical therapy in an effort to promote healing. With this added commitment the tension around the house was beginning to bubble over. With the calendar already full of appointments and activities an unexpected addition is not always a welcome part of the plan. We were committed to Lori's health so we made the necessary adjustments. We were exhausted by the end of each day and dropped into bed too tired to even catch up with each other on the day's events. We expended all our energy ensuring a smooth daily routine around the house and sometimes neglected seeking God's voice together. The physical therapy went on for a few weeks, but there really wasn't much of a change in Lori's ankle. In fact, it seemed like she was getting worse. She couldn't hold her foot up at all anymore and had to be careful that she didn't trip. We were both concerned and didn't understand why this was happening. We went back to the doctor and explained what was going on. He examined her again and decided to send her for tests.

One of the tests was an electric shock test called an electromyogram, or EMG. This was not a very pleasant test, but it showed the bad leg wasn't responding to the electrical currents shooting through her body. The test on the "good" leg showed the same. We were surprised at those results and knew then that we were dealing with something much bigger than just a sprained ankle, but we just didn't know what. A sense of confusion and anxiousness settled over us. We went home from those tests unsure of what the next step would be and uncertain of what was on the horizon.

The very next day, we spoke to the doctors about the results. The tests were inconclusive and they suggested we contact a specialist to further pursue causes, options and treatments. We called a neurologist immediately. Lori and I were both very surprised to find out we had to wait three weeks for an appointment. We really wanted to get in right away. But we had to wait. We refocused on the daily routine of the house while we waited for the appointment. This was for the kids sake as well as our own. We tried no to worry. Just under the surface, though there was a nagging feeling that something just wasn't right. Even with a strong faith in God, it is natural to feel anxious and unsure in the midst of difficulties you don't understand.

Finally, the day of our appointment arrived. The neurologist had a few ideas of what to look for, but nothing pointed to a definite cause for the lack of nervous response in Lori's legs. One of the diseases they tested for was Guillain -Barré syndrome. This is an uncommon disorder in which your own immune system attacks your nerves resulting in weakness and numbness that could eventually paralyze your entire body. These tests were very painful and difficult for Lori to endure and for me to watch. We both did our best to be strong. The EMG may have been the most painful. In this test needle electrodes are inserted into a muscle and an electric current goes through that muscle. Doctors are able to gather a lot of information from this test. An electrical impulse was sent from Lori's hip to her foot to determine if her weakness was due to muscle or nerve damage. She had to bite down on something and teared up during these tests. All I could do was hold her hand and pray. My prayers were taking on a new passion and intensity as the questions mounted and answers were elusive. We were becoming more and more anxious. My prayer life became less dignified and started to take on a twinge of desperation, which included a lot of "please" at the beginning and end of each request. I would have done anything to take that pain away from her. I felt so helpless. Yet, Lori was courageous, strong and in control even in these difficult circumstances. I admired her determination to get through each test.

When the hour of testing was over we went home to rest.

When I finally had a quiet minute to myself I was surveying everything that had happened in the past few months. Lori was struggling more each day to walk without tripping, the doctor visits had yielded no answers, and we had to wait three precious weeks for an appointment while Lori's condition continued to get worse. Why didn't anyone move faster or match our sense of urgency to do something helpful? We put our faith in doctors because they are trained to deal with sickness and disease, but it became clear to me that doctors have limited knowledge and power. I found myself very angry at the whole situation, at the doctors, and at the information vacuum in which we found ourselves.

During all of this Lori continued to work even as her condition continued to deteriorate. She was having some trouble with both legs and her hand control was also being affected. We started integrating a few pieces of helpful medical equipment into our daily lives. First, it was plastic braces on her lower legs and eventually she added a walker. She needed handles in the bathroom and shower to steady herself, and it wasn't long before she started using special utensils for eating. We prayed constantly that God would show up for us as Jehovah Rapha, the God who heals. We continued to believe He saw our situation and heard our prayers and He knew best.

As time went on, her mild paralysis began to have an effect on what she could do around the house. She had been accustomed to running things a certain way and taking care of the kids. Slowly she was becoming incapacitated and had to give up her expectation of how things would be at home. This was upsetting for her because she was use to taking charge. Losing control was the antithesis of how she was used to living her life. The dream we had envisioned so many years earlier at Longwood Gardens was moving further and further away. As Lori realized she was losing control it caused her to depend more and more on God for help and answers. This was not easy, but it was a forced necessity. She trusted that He would provide for her and for the family. Our faith became a matter of daily survival and we trusted our Heavenly Father to intervene in the situation. We were able to move ahead with confidence that He was with us each step of the way.

I saw my role for Lori and the family take on a new dimension as well. I came to terms with the fact that she was not able to do as much and took on more of the responsibilities around the house and in caring for the kids. I still had my pastoral and academic responsibilities too.

Life was very busy. I thought back to when Rachel was born and how I wanted to carefully protect my family. I felt a fresh surge of energy and passion to do whatever I could to protect them from this disease that had burst into our home. I firmly believed that we were in the midst of a battle, and I wanted to offer all of my strength to Lori and the kids. We read the bible and prayed together as much as possible. This was a huge source of encouragement for us and it kept our marriage strong. We had faith that God would heal Lori and we just had to be patient and wait for His perfect timing. The verses that came back to me over and over were from 2 Corinthians 4:

"We are pressed on every side by troubles, but we are not crushed. We are perplexed, but not driven to despair. We are hunted down, but never abandoned by God. We get knocked down, but we are not destroyed. Through suffering, our bodies continue to share in the death of Jesus so that the life of Jesus may also be seen in our bodies. That is why we never give up. Though our bodies are dying, our spirits are being renewed every day. For our present troubles are small and won't last very long. Yet they produce for us a glory that vastly outweighs them and will last forever! So we don't look at the troubles we can see now; rather, we fix our gaze on things that cannot be seen. For the things we see now will soon be gone, but the things we cannot see will last forever" (2 Corinthians 4:8-10;16-18).

I clung to Paul's reminder that we always need to look at our lives here on earth in view of eternity. There will be a day coming when time will have no meaning, and we will look back on our days upon the earth as just a moment. While living in the midst of suffering, it **feels** like an eternity, but Paul says it "won't last very long". You can only say that when God gives you an eternal perspective. Paul's life was anything but easy, but the Lord enabled him to think about the future in Glory that makes his suffering seem small and momentary. That's amazing!

In March 2002, our neurologist thought he had a diagnosis of Guillain-Barré syndrome. Lori needed prompt treatment by an eleven-day procedure called plasmapheresis. We were told that the majority of patients regain full functional capacity shortly after this procedure. Lori and I both believed that she would recover after this treatment with proper rest and physical therapy. We were getting to the point where we started bargaining with God for her health. We thought that we had gained all the wisdom there was to gain from the situation, that we had really learned a good lesson. Our character building exercise was complete and God could relieve us of this awful situation. It's common to want to cut a deal with God. He has his own agenda though and He is more interested in our character and holiness than He is in our comfort. It was getting harder and harder to pray like Jesus, "not my will, but your will be done."

Rachel, who was 12 at the time, came in to our room as we packed for the hospital that morning. She had gone through her Bible and wrote out encouraging verses and put them in a beautiful picture frame.

The three that blessed us most are:

> "The LORD your God is with you, he is mighty to save. He will take great delight in you, he will quiet you with his love, he will rejoice over you with singing." (Zephaniah 3:17)

> "For I am the LORD, your God, who takes hold of your right hand and says to you, do not fear; I will help you. Do not be afraid for I myself will help you," declares the LORD, your Redeemer." (Isaiah 41:13-14)

"I wait quietly before God, for my victory comes from him. He alone is my rock and my salvation, my fortress where I will never be shaken." (Psalm 62:1-2)

Who would have guessed God would reach out to us through a twelve year old, but that's whom He chose to deliver a message that day. We readily received the encouragement and kissed the kids goodbye.

We arrived at the hospital with nervous hope and after the usual admission procedures we finally got settled into a room. We prayed some more and held hands in anticipation of the outcome of the treatments. Eleven days was a long time to be in the hospital, especially when your only stay prior to that day was when you were born and when your children were born. Lori was always healthy, at least until recently. But we tried to make the best of a difficult situation. I worked hard and intentionally to make her smile and laugh. We watched sitcoms and had many visits from close friends. We embraced God's Word and believed God's promises. We also gained encouragement from reading about other people's faith.

One of the stories of faith that inspired us was the life of Fanny Crosby. Fanny was born to a poor family in Southeast, Putnam County, New York in 1820. When she was six weeks old, she caught a cold and developed inflammation of the eyes. The family physician was not available, and the man who came in his place recommended a hot, medicated cloth be placed over her eyes as a treatment. The botched procedure blinded her.

Life did not get easier. Her father died when she was one year old, so her mother and grandmother raised

her. Fanny was trained in extensive Bible memoriza-
tion and was a lifelong Methodist. She was incredibly
gifted in poetry and forever in love with her Savior. At
age eight she wrote this about her blindness:

> Oh what a happy soul I am,
> Although I cannot see;
> I am resolved that in this world
> Contented I will be.
> How many blessings I enjoy,
> That other people don't;
> To weep and sigh because I'm blind,
> I cannot, and I won't."

To this day, the vast majority of American hymnals con-
tain her work. Before her death, she had written over
8,000 hymns. She was very well known during her time
and often met with famous public figures including
presidents and military generals. She played the hymn
"Safe in the Arms of Jesus" at President Grant's funeral
in 1885. In her later years, she also became a popular
public speaker. She taught English and History in a
school for the blind in New York.

Why was she one of our heroes? Fanny accepted
her "disability" as a God-ability. I think it takes as
much, if not more, faith to accept your affliction as it
does to believe for your healing. Fanny once said, "It
seemed intended by the blessed providence of God
that I should be blind all my life, and I thank him for
the dispensation. If perfect earthly sight were offered
me tomorrow I would not accept it. I might not have
sung hymns to the praise of God if I had been distracted
by the beautiful and interesting things about me." She

also projected "when I get to heaven, the first face that shall ever gladden my sight will be that of my Savior!" Wow! What a faith! Lori and I wanted that same faith to trust that what was given to us was not a curse but a blessing.

Today I can honestly say that I am grateful to the Lord for all that we went through because I am a different man now, my faith is stronger, my peace is greater, and the way I minister to others in the face of adversity and grief is much more empathetic. Would I want to go through it all again? Absolutely not! But God had his purposes, and for that I praise Him.

Lori had never been in a hospital for an extended time so the lengthy stay was not easy for her. She was humbled by the constant attention and level of medical care she received from the nursing staff. Cards came pouring in from concerned friends and neighbors and I would sit and read to her the emails from my computer that greatly encouraged her spirit.

I still had responsibilities with the kids at home so I was torn between the hospital and home. Josh, especially, missed us both tremendously. Often, he would not sleep in his own bed because he was too lonely. He fell asleep in my bed and waited for me to come home. He missed Lori so much. Despite all this time by her bedside I missed her too. I missed life as it was before the illness; our walks through Longwood Gardens, our lunches at the local Chinese buffet restaurant and the unencumbered hugs we so freely exchanged. What I didn't miss though was her beauty because I saw it every moment of every day even in the pain. She battled every trial with grace and dignity because of God's grace and dignity working through her. Her beauty radiated from every cell of her person even through these difficulties. I loved her more deeply those days than any other in our 15-year marriage. I understood in a more practical and clear way the phrase "in sickness and in health". We were growing together in faith and were determined to trust God no matter what happened. We firmly believed that God would heal Lori. I was told a clever acronym for F.A.I.T.H. It's "Forsaking All I Trust Him". Lori and I could not place our faith on anything or anyone but the Lord. And we trusted Him completely. We continued to pray "come Jehovah Rapha with healing on your wings". We believed the verse in 1 Peter 2:24 was for us and we stood firmly on God's promise.

4

Lifted Up on Eagle's Wings

"Even when I walk through the darkest valley, I will not be afraid, for you are close beside me. Your rod and your staff protect and comfort me.

Psalm 23:4

After eleven long days in the hospital, we had high hopes for good news. We met with the doctor full of anticipation of the results of the treatment. The doctor did not deliver good news though. The procedure to treat Gulliane-Barré syndrome did not help. Our hopes were crushed. All of the time invested and all of those painful tests and this wasn't even Gulliane-Barre? I felt like were right back to square one again. Lori did not take the news well either. She tried so hard to remain positive. I could see her trying to will herself to walk with renewed energy. But it wasn't there. Every step she took was so difficult. We all were so desperate to see an improvement, but none came. Anger and frustration set in. We needed an answer about what was going on. Her condition was worsening every day and we still didn't have a diagnosis. We just continued to pray for a miracle. We wanted Lori to be physically well, but God had something much deeper in mind. God wanted to do a miracle in her soul, but we couldn't see that. We went home to rest and spend time with the kids.

We tried to keep a routine around the house and a focus on what the kids needed even though it was very difficult. We prayed with them about their schoolwork and whatever was on their minds. We tried to reassure them, calm their fear, and provide as much security as possible. We prayed with them for Lori's healing. She was still able to help the kids with their home-work, although she was frustrated with her inability to write neatly. We tried to lighten the mood with a little fun. Since Lori was more house bound than usual, we played board games and card games like Old Maid and Uno, and rented movies. It was good for both of us to be in the midst of the laughter that kids seem to naturally carry with them. We huddled together over the activity of the minute and tried to reconnect. We ran errands together since Lori could no longer handle this alone. Though the kids were impatient with the time it took to get Lori in and out of our mini-van, they enjoyed taking turns pushing her in the wheelchair. They especially liked large areas like the local mall since there was lots of space to maneuver and pick up speed. Luckily there were no accidents.

It wasn't long before we heard from the doctors. They finally sent us to the University of Pennsylvania hospital. Again, it was hurry and wait for the next appointment. Lori was glad to go home and spend time with the kids. We tried to keep life even and predictable while waiting for the next appointment. When we finally did meet with the doctors at the University hospital they wanted to re-run the very painful EMG. We were tired and weary. The thought of going through another round of long, painful tests weighed heavy on us. We needed answers though. Lori braved the tests and we waited again. The waiting may very well be the hardest part of the process. Every thought goes through your mind when there are unanswered questions. It is a time when your mind can overtake you if you let it. It was best to fill our minds and hearts with the Word of God and with song. So many evenings I would sit at the piano and play while Lori cleaned up and sang along. I loved to listen to her beautiful voice chime in with my keyboard. As the disease progressed Lori started to get frustrated because her speech was slurred and she couldn't keep up. She began to sound like a stroke victim, slurring her syllables into a garbled sound difficult to discern. But that never mattered to me or to the Lord. God looks at the heart (1 Samuel 16:7) and I believe that when God saw Lori's heart, He was very pleased.

Finally, we were called to the doctor's office for the diagnosis. It was May 9, 2002 when we sat down for the news. Getting bad news can be one of the hardest experiences that life has to offer. It very well may be one of the few forces on earth that actually stops time. The day of Lori's diagnosis was horrible. We sat huddled together in the office holding hands and bracing ourselves for the worst. The doctor said, "Lori, we have completed all the tests and we have confirmation: You have ALS. I'm sorry." Even though we were expecting bad news my mind still rejected hearing it. Random thoughts swirled as my brain tried to make sense of the diagnosis. We sat there stunned, unable to move. We weren't exactly sure what to do next. Do we just get up and go home? Do we demand to see results of tests? What just happened? Waves of emotion overtook us. I am sure our screaming and broken hearts echoed through the halls of heaven that day. "Is that it? You're sorry? What about treatment? Possible cures?" There were none. The dark shadows loomed in the office. It was a death sentence.

We walked out of the office that day a broken and emotional wreck. We instinctively did what we had always done. We turned toward the Lord for strength. We knew He would raise us up like on wings of eagles and He had not abandoned us. Even though the storm raged around us our roots went deep into the soil of God's love. We carried in our hearts the vision of heaven from the previous summer. God knew this was coming. God knew all along. News like that was an unbearable horror to us, but was not a horror to God. Through our tears and shock we clung to these truths for dear life.

It is probably hardest to trust God after receiving bad news. It yields confusion and anger, which sometimes can stamp out trust. When Lori and I received the proper diagnosis, I found the waves of anger crashing over my own soul. It went beyond frustration at the previous neurologist who kept coming up with the wrong analysis. I was angry that he did not suggest another specialist in Philadelphia that specializes in her symptoms. I was angry that it took several weeks of waiting in between appointments where we just literally sat around and worried. It's easy to forget God is in control of even all that. I didn't want to forgive that neurologist who I felt wasted months of our lives that we could have spent otherwise if we had only known Lori's sickness was fatal. I was hurt, furious and it felt justified. Jesus tells me to pray in Matthew 6:12 "...and forgive us our sins, as we have forgiven those who sin against us." That's a hard thing to pray. Someone once reminded me that when an individual sins against me, that offense was either already "paid for" on the cross (if that person is a true believer) or, one day, that person will pay the penalty for that offense against me along with every other sin they ever committed. Somehow God uses that to disarm my anger. Along with that, I try to remember how much I have been forgiven and also remind myself that the day is coming where God is going to right all wrongs and all the hurts of this world will be long forgotten as I get swept up in the beauty of my Savior face to face (1 Corinthians 13:12).

5

The Winds of Change

"With your unfailing love you lead the people you have redeemed. In your might, you guide them to your sacred home."

Exodus 15:13

We left the doctors office overwhelmed with uncertainty and grief. The shadow of death blanketed us as we walked out into the sunshine unsure of the future. Our hearts were churning. Verses filled my mind as I tried to find a way around this with God. I prayed based on 2 Kings 20. "Oh God you heard King Hezekiah's prayer for extended life. You answered that prayer Lord. You can answer it for us too can't you? You can extend Lori's life. Please answer that prayer for us too." I thought of Daniel 3:17-18. "Lord you saved Shadrach, Meshach, and Abednego from the flames. Surely you can save us from this fate as well. Please answer this prayer. Please save Lori." We had suspected all along that the diagnosis wasn't going to be what we wanted to hear. We still had the wind knocked out of us. Everyone knew we were going for the results that day and when Lori and I got into the car we knew we were going to have to tell people right away. We decided on a swift and direct approach. We actually made our first stop on the way home.

We stopped at Lori's boss's house, Russ. He was Lori's boss, but much more than that. He was like a father to her and he cared about Lori a lot. We broke the news to him and he cried and hugged Lori. He offered many prayers for her well being throughout the time she was sick and sent Lori little notes telling her so. Next we called Lori's family and drove out to Harrisburg to deliver the news in person. As expected this was not an easy visit. Tears of love flowed freely and the family pulled together as a stronghold of support for both of us. Their continued prayers were an inexhaustible source of strength.

Telling the children was maybe the hardest of all. We were unsure of how much to tell them. My son Josh was 9 at the time and had limited understanding of what exactly was going on. We tried to tell Rachel as much as we thought she needed to know, but not necessarily the entire story. However, in these days of Internet searches maybe giving her complete, accurate information would have been best. Young people today are information savvy and if they want to know something they can pretty much find it on the Internet. Rachel looked up the disease on line and did quite a bit of reading about it. She was angry when she found out we tried to keep information from her. Of course we only had her best interests in mind. We didn't have the clarity of thought that we normally would have given the situation. We worked it through with her and she did come to a complete understanding of what was happening.

After contacting immediate family and friends I sent this email out to our extended circle of friends.

Dear friends,

Today we found out that Lori has ALS. It is a disease that affects the motor neurons in the brain and spine. We are devastated by this news. We are looking at making several large changes in our lifestyle to accommodate Lori's needs. We appreciate your continued support and prayers. My concern is that Lori not be overwhelmed this week by too many calls from friends who want to help. We need a little time to grasp the immensity of what lies ahead and the most helpful thing right now is privacy and prayer. Pray for God's guidance and healing and strength. Lori will probably stop working soon and I need to decide if I can continue in seminary. We have a lot of adjustments ahead of us and at this point, we are pressing on and taking all this one day at a time. The Lord is changing us to become more like little children who trust without question. We are trusting him with our every need. Isn't that the way it is suppose to be? "Give us THIS DAY our daily bread". We plead with you all to intercede for us in this dark time that God would have mercy on us as a family.

In a way, the news was a relief. At least we knew what we were dealing with and what to expect. The scientific community is making progress on ALS research, but is still years away from a cure. Also known as Lou Gehrig's disease, as many as 30,000 Americans have the disease at any given time. It usually affects people between the ages of 40 and 70. Normally, most "PALS" (Patients of ALS) eventually lose ability to walk, use their arms, swallow and ultimately lose their ability to breathe. What was ahead was becoming clearer to us. Time became a dwindling resource but we tried not to dwell on the dismal prognosis, Instead we focused on what needed to be done to cope. Initially, this was easier said than done. I still couldn't believe that the whole situation was happening to us. I kept thinking, "She's only 37!" I was mad at the sickness, at her condition and for the time we wasted with tests that proved nothing. We made a conscious effort to focus on the responsibilities in front of us, and not waste time wallowing in anger. There was a lot of work to be done. I am sure God's grace surrounded us and strengthened us to move forward.

An immediate task was my job. In addition to the pastoral responsibilities at church, I was teaching piano through the local adult night school program to make some extra money. The day after receiving the news I had piano lessons to teach. Needless to say I was distracted during class. There were 12 students who were all on portable keyboards. The room was definitely too small and as I was attempting to reach out to one woman in the far corner of the studio, my left foot became lodged between two occupied piano benches. All six feet six inches of me went down and my foot twisted pretty hard. After three weeks of misdiagnosis, a second set of x-rays finally revealed a Lis Franc dislocation on the top of the foot above the big toe. Yesterday was an ALS diagnosis and today a broken foot! I cried out "God, this can't be happening to my family!" As the reality of our situation set in, so did the questions. The lost cries of desperation went up to God daily. "What are we going to do? Is God going to heal her? How are we going to provide everything she's going to need? How are we going to pay for everything? How can I take care of her when I am also temporarily disabled?

The truth in the situation is that God was never taken off guard. He didn't wake up one morning flustered and at a loss for what to do because of what He saw. He had his provisions waiting in the wings. The ALS Association in Philadelphia was our first blessing. They have a state-of-the-art facility and offer invaluable resources to ALS patients. We had an appointment set up for May 22 to meet with a top ALS neurologist, nursing staff, occupational therapist, social worker, psychologist and nutritionist all in one three hour visit. It sounded exhausting yet hopeful. We were glad to receive professional advice about the lifestyle changes that were coming. God's provision continued through Lori's grandmother who had a medical recliner that would lift Lori up to a standing or sitting position with the push of a button. A neighbor, whose mother had recently passed away, gave us a wheelchair that would make getting around the house easier. It also had a tray attachment so Lori could eat from the chair if she wanted to. With Lori using the wheelchair more, we traded in our two cars for a van that would transport her while sitting in the chair. By this time she was somewhere between using the leg braces and walker and using the wheelchair. Depending on the situation she used both to get around. Someone even donated a chair lift that would take Lori up and down the steps. The kids enjoyed riding the chair up and down the steps when she wasn't on it. Thank God for children who can create fun from any kind of situation.

With every piece of new equipment in the house there was an accompanying loss and adjustment. The day the wheelchair came into the house Lori looked at it and said, "I'll never get up from that chair again". The disease was taking not only a physical toll, but an emotional toll as well. Another big change looming in the near future was a decision about when Lori would quit her job. It was more and more difficult to move around and the decision seemed obvious. It was one more loss added to the long list of losses we had already experienced. These initial changes were difficult and we could hardly keep up. The new equipment in the house was overtaking our cozy living room. The wheelchair was bumping into walls. Use of the bathroom became harder. Lori was losing her ability to move her feet and legs faster than we expected. Each new item added to our house was a loss of the normal we had worked so hard to build. We had to give up control of so many expectations.

Even with the inevitable closing in, we focused as best we could on the immediate. We determined to make the most of the time we had and each day became a new gift. We did not want the time to be laden with depression and gloom, so we tried to focus on the fun we knew how to have. We wanted the time we had to be full of as many good memories as possible. The church had allowed me to take a leave of absence so that I could take care of Lori full time and it was a true blessing to be out from under the pressures of work. I didn't have to be out of the house by a certain time in the morning so Lori and I took the liberty to stay up late and talk and eat as much junk food as we wanted. I also remember watching a lot of television. The TV provided an excuse for a mental break. Our favorite show was "Whose Line Is It Anyway". Although sometimes inappropriate for prime time TV we loved the spontaneity of the program. I always looked for the humorous stuff on TV because it had a way of just lightening the load. Laughter is such good medicine for the soul.

One night, as we were flipping channels and trying to relax, the conversation turned toward what we wanted to do with the time we had left. The idea of going to Disney World came up. It sounded crazy, but we were young and still very much in love and we decided that it was a good idea. We didn't think family and friends would be too supportive, but we firmly made up our minds to take the kids to Disney. We wanted to make good memories for them and we didn't have much time. So we booked the trip for June and allowed the anticipation to redefine the mood in our house. I really couldn't walk since breaking my foot, but we had an adventure laid out before us and we embraced it. Some of the women from the church bible study helped us make the arrangements and before we knew it the day arrived and off we went. Lori was in her wheelchair and I was in mine. The two kids were right beside us. I don't know how we made it through the airports and to the hotel, but we did. The week was perfect. We did all we could at Disney. The two wheelchairs gave us rights to the front of every line. We had a great time bypassing the hour or more wait for whatever attraction we were getting on. We made it through the park in no time. The whole family had a great time. Lori was very tired most days, but she was determined to enjoy herself. For a short time the Florida sunshine seemed to chase away the foreboding shadows and we were free to just enjoy life again. However, as we all know, vacations have a bad habit of coming to an end and this vacation was no different.

6

O Little Church of Bethlehem

"Let us hold unswervingly to the hope we profess, for he who promised is faithful. And let us consider how we may spur one another on toward love and good deeds."
Hebrews 10:23-24

We often wonder exactly where God is when we are facing the storms of life. It sometimes feels like dark clouds cover his face. Just as we are assured that the sun exists behind threatening storm clouds we can also have full confidence that God exists in the midst of threatening situations in life. Do you know where? He's in His people. God shows Himself most clearly through the body of Christ. The members of Bethlehem United Methodist church were living examples of how God moves on earth. While we were in Florida a caring crew donated their time and energy for a week to transform our home into a wheelchair friendly place. The doorways were enlarged, more handles were installed in the bathroom, the downstairs bathroom was expanded and adjustments were made to our bedroom and bed. Their example of selfless service stands to this day as a shining example of God's love in action. When we arrived home from Florida and came through the front door we had mixed feelings about our "new" home. We were overcome with the dedication and obvious hard work that so many people had put in to make the house more wheel chair friendly. These much-needed changes provided a welcomed relief from the physical restrictions with which we had previously dealt. At the same time, they were another profound loss, even though they needed to be done. We worked so hard to buy the house and make it a home. Even our home was now permanently changed because of this disease. There was no aspect of our lives that was untouched.

God showed us over and over again how He can reach out to us through people. It was a blessing to us as well as to the people who were giving. For example, God worked through my friend, Glenn, who gave us the chair lift that Lori used to get up and down the stairs. God worked through Elaine and Donna who came over and cleaned up breakfast and made lunch. Elaine's husband, Ed, installed a handrail in one of our bathrooms. God worked through Heidi and her Bible Study small group who helped us plan the trip to Florida. God worked through Jim and Tom who built a ramp outside the front door so Lori could safely get in and out of the house. Serving doesn't sound very glamorous, but it is very fulfilling.

God worked through Pastor Jon who stopped by and encouraged us tremendously. He told us that our attitude is that of Paul in Romans 14:7-9. "For none of us lives to himself alone and none of us dies to himself alone. If we live, we live to the Lord; and if we die, we die to the Lord. So, whether we live or die, we belong to the Lord. For this very reason, Christ died and returned to life so that he might be the Lord of both the dead and the living." God worked through Linda, Cindy, Scott, Tricia, Mike, Sue, Helen, Eileen, Joy, Irene, Debbie, Matt, and the countless people who have brought us meals, gifts, housecleaning, cards and phone calls. This was how God chose to make his presence known to us, through others. Combine these gestures of love with the Holy Spirit, His peace and comfort, and we found both hope and endurance.

I want to offer a balance to the idea of allowing people to help. There are a lot of well-intentioned people who want to do something during a time of crisis. You have to pick and choose the times that are convenient for you. There are times that "help" isn't very helpful. There may be a personal matter to deal with or the person who is sick may feel exceptionally run down and unable to talk to a lot of people that day. There are all kinds of reasons why you may not want a lot of people involved on a certain day. We were thankful for the help and concern people showed, but we also coveted our personal space. We handled this by putting a sign on the front door, "Lori doesn't feel well today. Please do not knock or come in if this sign is posted on the door". We explained to our friends in advance that we weren't trying to be rude and we weren't ungrateful for their help, but we did need a way to communicate to them that we needed family time.

Even with all the help we received it became clear that we needed someone with us full time. God's provision was the clearest through Lori's mom, Bonnie. After some prayer and discussion we decided to ask her to stay with us and help with Lori's care, the house and kids. Bonnie chose to quit her job and move in to help full time with whatever Lori needed. A mom's heart is tireless, determined and fierce. I was thankful for the strength she brought to a difficult situation. We moved Bonnie in and she spent the summer helping me with Lori's daily care, and the chores around the house. We both savored each precious day we had. The disease continued to progress quickly and it seemed like with each passing day Lori grew weaker. Along with the physical difficulties there were emotional difficulties to deal with. How do you face the fact that you're dying? How can you wrap your mind around that thought without going totally crazy? We dealt with this through many nights of tears and pain. It was exhausting. We would have a time of grieving and crying and then muster our strength to tackle the next day's activities and responsibilities. We tried to spend time reading and praying together every day. We also used the time to talk about whatever pressing issue was at hand.

One of the items we discussed during our time together was what Lori could leave for the children. She wanted to leave something for the kids so that she could be a part of the special events of their lives and let them know how much she loved them. Getting to the point of doing something was not easy. We had talked about it previously but she resisted the idea because she had not yet come to terms with the inevitable reality of the children's future. She finally came to the point where she was ready to move ahead. Lori worked *very* hard putting together gifts for the future. She and I went through every piece of her jewelry and earmarked each one that the kids would get at different milestones of their lives. For instance, Lori was a swimmer and in her teen years had received a medal in a swim competition. She had me set aside that medal for the day when Josh would learn how to swim. Earrings would be given to Rachel once she was brave enough to get her lobes pierced. Knowing that some of Rachel's taste in jewelry was different than her own, we went shopping together for necklaces and rings that would be suitable to wear. By the time we finished we had gifts set aside for the kids for every Christmas, many birthdays and other special events. I have them all hidden deep in my closet. As painful as it is to pull that box out, there is an aspect to it that makes it feel like Lori is rejoining the family on Christmas and on the children's birthdays.

In addition to the gifts there are also voice recordings that were made for the children. One day she even attempted to make a video recording for the family, but staring into that camera and talking was just too emotional. Up to that moment, I had never seen Lori cry so hard in my life. But after that, when she was alone and still able to maneuver the laptop with one working finger, she did several voice recordings, for certain milestones in the kid's lives. These recording are true gifts of love and treasures to the children. Although very emotional, Lori was able to create a voice recording for me as well. In addition to words of love she reminds me that each child is in constant need of hugs and should be told daily that they are loved. I have treasured that CD and it has been played many times over the years.

These acts of love are such terrific examples of how to make the most of every day. I'm not saying it's easy or that it comes without a lot of tears, but it was her ministry to her family based on what she could do. She used the time to focus on giving to the people she cared about. She did not allow the disease that was taking over her body to take over her spirit too but rather continued to serve God as faithfully as possible.

Finally, the end of the summer was upon us and we took one more trip. We went to the Jersey shore for a week and stayed at a Christian retreat and vacation place. I was able to take Lori and the kids to the beach. We played games together and we rested our souls. There is something healing about the beach. We took in as much of the ocean air as possible and tried to slow time to a halt. If X marks the spot for the hidden treasure, it must have been right under our beach chairs because our last vacation together was golden.

7

"Jesus wept"

John 11:35

Before we knew it September was upon us again. I thought back to the previous September when we were in the Poconos with the family. Lori tripped that day and sprained her ankle. I shook my head in disbelief as I thought of everything we had been through in a year. To everyone's disappointment the days started getting shorter. The long shadows cast off the horizon were more obvious as they stole away the remaining minutes of precious sunlight. Autumn reminds us each year that although we fight against death, the process of dying can be very beautiful if done under the guiding hand of God. Just look at how He directs the trees each year. Their leaves die off in a brilliant splash of color that is magnificent to see. People make special plans to go out and watch how God directs this most awesome change from life to death. He does not leave nature to itself. He himself is the grand director of each move the earth makes. If He takes the time to direct birth and death in nature how much more can He play an intimate role in the birth and death of his beloved children if we allow him to be a part of the process? God wants to be included in each step, but He won't force himself. He always waits for an invitation.

Lori did invite Him to be a part of her process and she relied on His strength for so many difficult transitions. One transition was the process of letting go of the kids. Lori realized that as time went on she would become more incapacitated and unable to speak. She knew she had limited communication time to accomplish a very big task for them. She had to step back more and let me take over the areas that she normally would have attended to. The one example that stands out was an evening when Rachel was in an argument with me over a trivial matter. Lori, lying in bed but fully alert to all that was going on around her, was trying to communicate her disapproval over how I was handling Rachel. By this time, she talked with a severe slur and I really could not understand what she was saying. I couldn't even hand her a white-board or computer because she had no use of her hands. Without any success, Lori looked at me as if she was going to growl like a mama bear. Her eyes were filled with frustration. All of the sudden, she bowed her head with her chin resting squarely on her chest. I waited to see what would happen next. A few minutes later, her head popped up just as fast as it had gone down. She fixed her eyes on me and with a surprisingly clear tone she said, "I did it". "You did what?" I questioned. With tears welling up in her eyes, she replied, "I gave you up...all of you. I no longer have the capacity to run this family.

They are your responsibility now. I just can't do it". I believe that I was watching her surrender a part of herself she had held on to for so long. She gave up her need to control. Romans 8:28 states, "And we know that in all things God works for the good of those who love him, who have been called according to his purpose." Lori's sickness, although horrible, was actually the refining fire of God. What Satan meant for evil God used for her good. She learned through her sickness how to relinquish faith in her own ability and to trust God with everything that was dear to her right down to her husband, her children, and her very own life. She realized what was true all along. God is really the one in charge; He is the one who has control over each of us if we yield our lives to him. She realized that He would take care of her every need, my every need and everything the children needed. She was forced to give up control of her body, but she willingly relinquished control of her spirit to God. This process played out in a very dramatic way and serves as a vivid reminder to all of us that we too are in the same process of learning to relinquish control of our lives to God. Each of us is in a unique situation, but God requires the same from everyone, total trust in Him.

Through the process God does not abandon us. He reminds us regularly that even as we endure the pain that life inflicts He wants to be intimately involved in our suffering. This was illustrated beautifully one morning at church. Most Sundays it was very difficult for Lori to go to church. It was very difficult for her to see her friends all at once and most terminally ill people need time for themselves and their thoughts. Sometimes too much attention just increases stress already hidden deep inside. The process of letting go is very difficult and exhausting. By this time she needed a tremendous amount of care and getting her from the house to her place at church was monumental. Some days it was better to stay home but on this day we made it. Lori was sitting peacefully in her wheelchair enjoying the service. After the service, a kind gentle-looking man came up to her, knelt down at the foot holdings of her wheelchair and wept bitterly. After a couple of moments, he stood up without a word and left the building. It was quite peculiar at the moment, but even more when he did not attend another Sunday morning until I brought Lori back to church a few weeks later. Once again, this gentle fellow dressed simply in a clean flannel shirt and blue jeans, sat in the second to last pew on the right with his hands in his pockets. He waited until the service was over only to repeat what he had done before: fell to Lori's feet, wept and then left.

At a staff meeting two days later I asked if anyone noticed this gentleman in the back of the 10:30 service. Between the five or six members in attendance at that meeting I was the only one who had seen him. Bethlehem Church was averaging 250 people on Sunday mornings and the pastors were always keeping an eye out for newcomers. It was frustrating at the time knowing I couldn't even catch his name.

I could not get Lori back to church the following week, but we did finally go back a few weeks later. It was on a day I happened to be preaching on "Suffering". Guess who was sitting in the second to last back pew? It was the stranger again! As I stepped into the pulpit I thought, "This time I will get to that man before he exits the door." As it turned out the Holy Spirit moved in a very powerful way that morning and when the service finished, I had too many people lined up to talk with me. I could not get to Lori or the stranger. After 15 minutes or so, I finally came face to face with Lori and her big, beautiful brown eyes were like flowers dripping water after a refreshing rain. "He showed up again, didn't he?" I said, and all Lori could do was smile and give an affirmative nod.

When we returned home that morning my curiosity finally got he best of me and I just had to ask the question. "Who do you think that man is who keeps crying at your feet?" Without a moment of hesitation she declared, "I know he's an angel". This was the 4th time she had been visited by an angel. My theological mind was whirling. I asked her, "If that man really is an angel, and, according to the Bible, angels are God's messengers, then what's the message?" Lori, gazed at me from the wheelchair, with tears rolling down hers cheeks, quoted the shortest verse found in the Bible "Jesus wept" (John 11:35). At that point, that's exactly what I did. We both realized that God wanted to find a way to communicate a very powerful message about His love for us. It is my prayer that Christians everywhere take encouragement from this message. God sees your suffering. He knows how you feel. He cries when you cry and He is with you every step of the way. That was Lori's last visit to church. She was just too sick to return to the services.

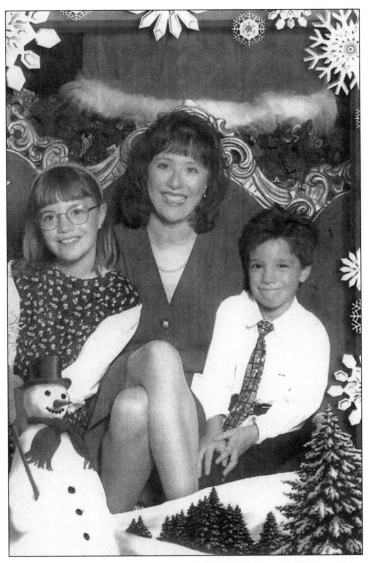

Lori took the kids to the mall to take a family picture
to give me as a Christmas gift and was frustrated
that she couldn't find a store available. Angry and
desperate, she told Santa to step aside, 'cause she was
getting a family picture done...and he's not part
of the family!

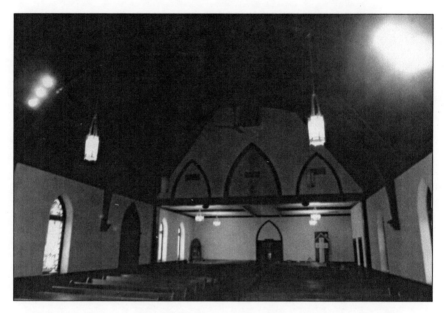

The rafters of Bethlehem Church where Lori saw
angels dancing in a circle shortly before her first ankle
injury in 2001.

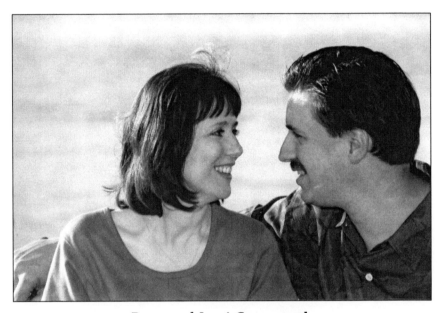

Dan and Lori Gottwerth
Last vacation together
Harvey Cedars, NJ

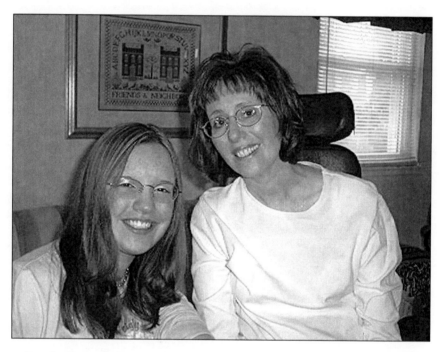

Rachel with Lori shortly before her death. Together,
Rachel learned how to stand up for her beliefs and
learn what Christian womanhood was all about. Lori
had a peace that Rachel was "going to be O.K." after
her death and that she had left a permanent mark in
Rachel's life.

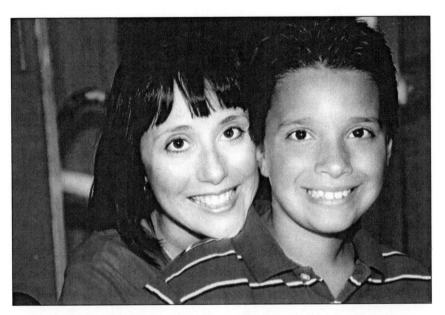

Lori with Josh. Josh was her "little dude". Josh always made Lori smile and they spent a ton of time just cuddling on the couch. Leaving the children without a mother was the sole reason that Lori hesitated about dying and going to Heaven. She didn't want to cause that kind of pain...for any of us.

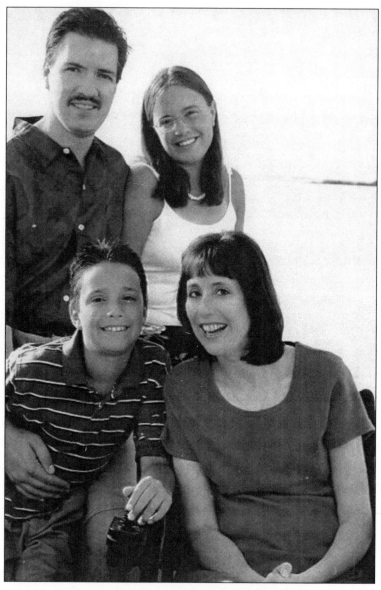

Lori, Rachel, Josh and myself at
Harvey Cedars Bible Conference
Long Beach Island, NJ

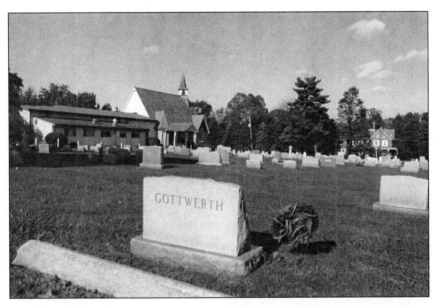

Lori's headstone resting at home with what was at that time our spiritual family—Bethlehem United Methodist Church in Thornton, PA

8

Unconditional Love

*"Your love for one another will prove
to the world that you
are my disciples."*
John 13:35

Thanksgiving that year was a blessing. What can be better than family gathered for a delicious meal? We really enjoyed the day and made it a point to thank God for all the blessings He had given us. Even with a foreboding feeling in the backs of our minds there was so much to be thankful for. He had revealed Himself to us in so many ways throughout the entire process. Lori wrote a letter that year to the family, in which she stated everything for which she was thankful. She was thankful that the disease taught her to be less task oriented and more people oriented. She was thankful to realize that the only things that really matter in life God provides for us. She was thankful for Jesus and how He made a way for us to get into heaven because of His tremendous love for us. She said she was not afraid of dying and carried with her the assurance of salvation.

As the chill of December settled in on us, I labored hard under the burden of care that was needed. Physically, I was wearing down. Even with Bonnie in the house to help I was still exhausted. Lori's condition was very bad. She labored under the burden of paralysis and she was exhausted as well. I had to carry her up and down the stairs each morning and evening. She lost all movement in her legs and hands and her arms weren't far behind. Her speech was very slurred and it was getting more and more difficult every day to understand her. This has to be one of the greatest frustrations for people with ALS. The body breaks down and the muscles give out but reasoning skills and alertness remain as sharp as ever. It is very hard and exhausting. I knew I should do something to take care of my own self as well. People often say, "Take care of yourself too. You're no good to anyone if you're burned out". That is true, but the reality is that there isn't much time to do anything for yourself. You should try to get out as much as your situation allows but when the demands of constant care take over try to be creative and find ways to take care of your own soul right in the house. I tried to find refuge and strength in the small aspects of life. There are plenty of activities that can serve as a source of refreshment. A sitcom on the television, a cup of coffee and a good book, a work out in the basement, a walk around the neighborhood or a quiet chat with a friend can all serve as sources of refreshment.

I tried to adjust my own attitude and enjoyed being with Lori in new ways. We read the Bible together a lot. We especially enjoyed the stories about the heroes of the faith. We learned through these stories about other people's struggles and how God helped them grow through each struggle. We realized that we weren't the first to go through a difficulty and many after us would experience the same. We were encouraged by these stories and drew strength from other's insights. We had given up dinners out a long time before, but there was a night when I hired a team to provide dinner in. We had sent the kids to friend's houses and Lori and I enjoyed gourmet cooking complete with a cello serenade right in our own living room.

Our marriage continued to grow stronger and she was as beautiful to me as ever. I took pleasure in learning to do for her what she couldn't do for herself anymore. I learned to apply mascara, pluck eyebrows and shave legs. I learned to give sponge baths, brush teeth and get her dressed. These may seem like menial tasks but to someone who is sick they are very important. At least when she looked in the mirror she saw her same beautiful face and not the devastation of her disease. Looking pretty helped her maintain some dignity. We turned these personal grooming experiences into a new kind of intimacy between us. We embraced the experiences as a new way to strengthen our marriage rather than a chore that needed to be checked off the list. I am glad no one was lurking with a camera outside the door because the sight of me trying to apply mascara to someone else would have been comic material for a long time to come. One day as I was helping her, she looked at me with tears in her eyes and said, "I'm so sorry that I have nothing to give back to you." I said to her, "Sweetheart, you have given me everything ever since the day you sat down in that wheelchair. You have shown me how to serve without expectation of or focus on what I will receive in return. You have taught me what unconditional love really means." This was a true gift to me because it enabled me to have a deeper understanding of how God loves.

I continually sent out email updates to friends and family. They were extremely concerned and bulk email was a great way to communicate. Apparently, one of my emails found its way to Joni Eareckson Tada. God never ceased to amaze us through this whole experience. Never in all my life would I have expected one of my emails to make it to Joni, but it did. God reached out to us once again through her to encourage us. Joni read the email and was inspired by the story. She actually wrote a beautiful letter of encouragement to Lori. She told us that she had heard about Lori's struggle with ALS and was praying for us. She shared some very relevant Scripture and enclosed some literature and a CD to encourage us. Our spirits were lifted through her correspondence and we were reminded once again that God was intimately involved with our situation.

Christmas came around and Bonnie and I tried to make the time festive and happy for the whole family. The shopping got done as it usually does and the preparations were made to the best of our ability. This was not an easy time but we just willed ourselves to have fun. Lori was still getting visits from close friends and Christmas was no exception. Sometimes the visits were difficult because she had less control over her emotions. This is a common experience for ALS patients. What would normally be overlooked and brushed off became an emotional disaster. She cried easily and had no way of stopping herself. This just added to the exhaustion she was already feeling and made it harder for others as well. Christmas is an emotional time anyway and this aspect of the disease just added to the difficulty. In spite of it all, we did our best to enjoy the time, the kids, and our family and friends.

9

Welcome Home

"The master said, 'Well done, my good and faithful servant. You have been faithful in handling this small amount, so now I will give you many more responsibilities. Let's celebrate together!'
Matthew 25:23

After Christmas Lori's condition had deteriorated so badly that we finally called hospice for some help and a hospital bed was set up in our bedroom. For the first time we were sleeping in a bed that wasn't our own. This was a profound loss for both of us. The marriage bed is set apart by God as a sanctuary between two people. It is not a place for outsiders. It is a source of rest, peace, renewal, refreshment, and intimacy. Although the bond between us was strong, this change reinforced in another tangible way the fact that what we had was slowly slipping away. Now instead of a sanctuary and a place of rest there was a strange bed and people we didn't know. This took an emotional toll on both of us.

The nurses were an invaluable strength in providing care for Lori. They administered daily medications to make her more comfortable and assisted with some of the difficult tasks that come with end of life care. During the month of January she became totally paralyzed and was hardly able to talk anymore. Her breathing became labored as the disease began its final assault.

Finally, the day came we had all been dreading. It was February 14th, 2003. I knew it would be our last Valentine's Day together as man and wife, but I had no idea that it was the last *full day* that we would ever spend together. Lori was able to communicate to her mom that she wanted her to go to the store and pick out a nice Valentine's card for me. Bonnie went right away to get this done for Lori, she signed the card on Lori's behalf and we exchanged our cards in the morning. It was a sweet time together. The rest of the day we proceeded through our normal routine until early afternoon when, Lori said something to me that caught me off guard. "Dan, I know you are going to fall in love again and eventually get remarried. I have told the kids that their father will be *pathetic* living alone and they will need to allow you to remarry". And with that statement she was able to give me a wink that always let me know that she was speaking the truth in love. She continued, "But Dan, even when you remarry, will you still... will I be...?" She either could not come up with the right words or just didn't want to say them. I took her hand and said "Lori, whomever that woman will be and whenever that will happen, you are and will always be, my first love. There is a part of me that will be taken to Heaven with you and I am going to love you forever." At that point, we both began to cry. From the moment I laid eyes on that beautiful woman almost 20 years earlier, I couldn't imagine looking at another woman the same way, much less getting married again. Trying to imagine either of us going through life without the other was just more than our hearts could bear.

The rest of that day was no different than others in that season of life. I tried to keep her comfortable, laughing and peaceful. Rachel was at a youth retreat with Bethlehem Church's youth group 45 minutes away. That evening as Lori's mother and I were getting her ready for bed, I could tell she was more restless than normal. Eating was nearly impossible without choking, so I went out to the local convenience store and picked up a large Slurpee for Lori's dinner. She managed to drink, and even enjoy, most of it. Sleeping that night was unusually difficult for her as well. I have heard it said on more than one occasion that those who are about to pass into eternity often do not sleep for a day or two before they go. It certainly was true of Lori. Despite the stresses and exhaustion of another challenging day Lori was up all night. It was as if she drank two liters of caffeine. Bonnie and I rotated the night shift and kept her amused and occupied as she lay next to me in our queen-sized hospital bed. I dozed off frequently but was awakened abruptly each time I realized she wasn't sleeping at all.

The following morning was the 15th of February. It had snowed during the night and was still coming down that morning when we took Lori downstairs. When Bonnie and I took her into the bathroom her face began to turn purple. I froze. I didn't know what to do. Bonnie quickly suggested that we put Lori into the recliner and as soon as we got her there, we noticed the color returning to her face. I knelt beside the recliner, looked deeply into her eyes and asked her, "Is this it?" I'm not sure why I asked *her*, but her reply was unmistakable. She nodded affirmation with as much confidence that she could muster. We both knew she was going home that day. I prayed, "God, what do I do?" My mind reeled with details. I had to get Rachel home. I had to call Pastor Jon. I made both of those calls immediately and then told Lori to hang on; Rachel was on her way.

ALS was taking its final blow on Lori's life. The disease had worked up from her feet and had made its way to her diaphragm, the final stop. I thought I was prepared for this day, but you are never *fully* prepared. I kept telling Lori how much I loved her. I woke Josh up and told him that Mom was going home to be with Jesus. He accepted it in a true childlike way, not fully understanding the extent of the ramifications.

Pastor Jon arrived first. He was surprised at how well Lori looked under the circumstances. He proceeded to talk to each family member to see how we were coping with what was happening. A few minutes later Rachel walked in with Tom and Cindy, Bethlehem Church's youth ministers. Lori was struggling to keep her diaphragm going, but I am convinced that the Lord gave her the *choice* to hold on to her life for a brief time. After taking a deep breath, she managed to communicate to Rachel these simple words: "*I love you and I am so proud of you*". Rachel needed to hear those words. Lori deeply loved Rachel and literally with her dying breath communicated that message of unconditional love and delight in her only daughter. She took extra time with Josh as well to make sure that he knew exactly how much she loved him and how proud she was of him.

Pastor Jon suggested that we pray together and as I sat next to Lori with my head in her lap listening to his prayer of surrender and child-like trust, something inside of me burst open like a dam. The past year and a half of being the strong one, the funny one, the composed one, just fell apart. I wept in a way that Lori had not seen in a very long time—certainly not since her diagnosis. And though I certainly didn't anticipate or desire that display of emotion, I think Lori needed to see it before she went home. Amidst my bitter anguish, I could hear a sigh of contentment rising out of the little breath that she had left. It almost felt like she was telling me to let it out, and that everything was going to be OK. I couldn't control myself. The river of pain and sorrow was beyond words. We had worked so hard together to make it through this illness, to keep her happy, comfortable, and positive and to keep the family together. Today, though, it was all over. It was time for her to go home to Jesus. Our days as husband and wife were complete. I had to say good-bye. As hard as I tried to prepare for this day, I just wasn't ready to let go.

After the prayer, I couldn't open my eyes for the longest time, afraid of allowing time to proceed. When I finally did open them, I found I was alone with Lori. Everyone else had moved into other rooms in the house. I looked up at her and what I saw is hard to put into words. Her eyes were as big as I had ever seen them, and she was staring across the room. For the life of me, I could not figure out what she saw, but it was obvious there was something supernatural that was being revealed to her. There have been countless stories told about an aspect of Heaven being uncovered for those about to cross over, and it is even backed up biblically with the account of Stephen in Acts 7:54-56. I am convinced that the gates of Heaven itself had been presented to her, and that the angel who had fallen at her feet at Bethlehem Church had come back to walk her into Glory. Can I prove it? No. But she saw something or someone that made her completely peaceful. "You will keep in perfect peace all who trust in you, all whose thoughts are fixed on you!" (Isaiah 26:3). God was so good to Lori, right to the very end.

Soon after that, Lori asked me to do something but as she struggled to communicate with me, her breath was so shallow that I couldn't understand her. After about 5 minutes of trying, I came to the conclusion that she was saying two words and the second word was "me". The first word was one syllable, but it took almost 10 very long minutes of trying to understand her before I finally realized the word was "hold". Hold me. Lori wanted me to hold her. I quickly wrapped my arms around her frail body, as she lay there paralyzed on the recliner. I told her that I loved her and that everything was going to be all right. Suddenly, I realized that she was trying to shake her head sideways as if to say "no!" I pulled away to look at her once again and asked her what's wrong. After all, I held her as tight as I could without crushing her. As I made eye contact with her, we made a connection heart to heart, man to wife, best friend to best friend. Though it could no longer be audible, I heard her loud and clear. "Sweetheart, pick me up in your arms, let me rest my head on my favorite spot in the cleft of your shoulder, and hold me until Jesus takes me". All of that was communicated by one last simple "hold me". Without another thought, I gently picked up her up for the last time. I thought of the "false alarm" of sorts a couple of weeks before. Then, too, she had asked me to pick her up and hold her. Like everything in her life, she knew exactly what she wanted at the time of death. When she died, she wanted to be in the place where she felt the most at home, the safest place—the nook of my left shoulder. Why was I surprised? She had planned it all. Not just for her, but for me.

After a several minutes, my arms began to grow weak from carrying her, so I sat on the sofa to rock her to her final sleep. I wanted to sing to her, and the only song that came to me in those last few moments together was the song "Breathe". I have no idea how that one popped into my head, but ironically (or not), the two things that will take away the life of an ALS patient is their ability to eat and their ability to breathe. How fitting were these words sung through a watershed of tears:

> This is the air I breathe, this is the air I breathe
> Your holy presence living in me
> This is my daily bread, this is my daily bread
> Your very Word spoken to me
> And I, I'm desperate for You
> And I, I'm lost without You

I sang that song over and over until I realized that Lori's breathing had ceased. She told me weeks before that she was not afraid of dying, but she but was afraid of how she would die. She did not want to struggle to breath or swallow. God was gracious to her and not only was she peaceful, but there was no struggle whatsoever. She was finally home with her Savior.

I quickly called out to my mother-in-law, Bonnie, and she came in and confirmed that Lori was gone. What happened next will live in my memory forever. There arose from deep in my soul a cry that I never knew was possible. I remember hearing Bonnie tell the kids "go to your Father". I felt the kid's arms touching me but all I could do was wail. It was horrible. I lost my best friend, and I just wanted to die with her.

I sat on that sofa with Lori cradled in my shoulder for over an hour. The funeral home was contacted but they were in the midst of a service so their arrival was delayed. This turned out to be a blessing to me because it allowed some closure to happen right there in my living room. Pastor Jon prayed a powerful prayer asking the Lord to enable me to turn Lori over to His loving hands. Bonnie had enough composure to send the kids to their bedrooms a couple of minutes earlier when people from the funeral home finally arrived. They assisted me in laying her on the gurney and I got a quick glance at her face. It wasn't her. Though her eyes were partly open, it wasn't my Lori. She really was gone. Even seeing that she wasn't there I still didn't want to let her go. As the hearse drove away from the house, it suddenly dawned on me that Lori would never grace our home with her presence again. She was not coming back; she had a new home. I had never felt so alone.

10

Looking Forward

"Oh, that we might know the Lord! Let us press on to know him. He will respond to us as surely as the arrival of dawnor the coming of rains in early spring."
Hosea 6:3

The final task before me was the funeral. Like everything else about her illness, Lori had ideas about how she wanted it to be, and left specific instructions. One request was that no one show up in black, but instead wear brightly colored clothing to acknowledge that she was home and free. It was important to her to honor God in the service as well as give people a chance to say their final good-byes. We also planned for a time of worship. Funerals are never easy to get through and this one was no different, but in the end we honored Lori and we honored God.

The kids and I spent time together grieving in the months that followed. We needed each other, and stuck very close together. At times it felt like living a dream.

When one is forced to endure the unbearable, has created us with an amazing capacity to comp sate. Your brain allows you to forget the whole t for a short time, and then like a freight train the re comes barreling through. You are once again o whelmed with pain and a multitude of emotion; g loss, anger, brokenness. But even the deepest of e tions are not too much for the Lord. I leaned heavily on the Him during this time. He is always there to comfort us in our time of need and I let his Word flow freely through my heart. As I reflected on all these events the Lord revealed to me several truths that now anchor my heart to his.

1. God is never late and never early, He is always right on time.

In the initial stages of grief it's common to ask why. Why him/her? Why this way? Why now? Why at this age? Who can understand all of God's decisions? The answers to 'why' for some questions may exist only on the other side of death. We can stand on the rock of this truth though: God's timing is perfect. I have seen this over and over. God tends to reveal His will and answers to our prayers only after much waiting and heart-wrenching prayer on our part. Why would He do that? Does He like to see us agonize and worry? Absolutely not! On the contrary, the Lord does *not want us* to worry and fret. (Matthew 6:25-34; Mark 13:11; Matthew 13:22; Philippians 4:6; 1 Peter 5:7). The Lord wants us to wait patiently for Him. Character development often comes in the waiting. When the Apostle Paul battled with a message from Satan, he prayed on three different occasions over a period of time before

God answered him, and even then God didn't give him the answer he wanted to hear. That thorn in his flesh remained for the rest of his life (see 2 Corinthians 12:1-10). God will never be late when answering our prayers, but He is rarely "early" by our definition. Our attitude should be that of Micah: "As for me, I look to the Lord for help. I wait confidently for God to save me, and my God will certainly hear me." (Micah 7:7)

2. God turns misery into ministry

"All praise to God...who comforts us in all our troubles so that we can comfort others. When they are troubled, we will be able to give them the same comfort God has given us. For the more we suffer for Christ, the more God will shower us with his comfort through Christ. Even when we are weighed down with troubles, it is for your comfort and salvation! For when we ourselves are comforted, we will certainly comfort you. Then you can patiently endure the same things we suffer. We are confident that as you share in our sufferings, you will also share in the comfort God gives us" (2 Corinthians 1:3-7).

Not only does God use our trials to make us holy, He also uses them to help encourage other Christians in their walk with Christ. It's all part of the way God redeems brokenness. "This book you hold in your hands is the result of the most painful and trying time of my life. But God has chosen to use those agonizing circumstances to benefit others. It brings a lot of joy to my heart to know that Lori's suffering served a bigger purpose. Likewise, your pain and suffering is not just for your benefit, but it is to benefit other Christians in their walk and to lead non-Christians to a personal relationship with Jesus Christ.

3. God is Good

In spite of life's hardships and trials, God is on the throne and He is good! He loved us so much that He sent His only Son into the world to die a death we should have died, to make a way for us to enter into His heaven and enjoy Him forever. It may be hard to believe in the face of the most miserable kind of suffering that God is good, but it is true. It's only when we lose sight of his role in our story that life seems dark, foreboding and cruel. If we welcome him into the story He will shine his light on the most horrible suffering and turn it into a strength, a victory, an instrument of refinement for our soul and an example of his love to all.

4. The "valley of the shadow of death" is just a path to higher ground

"Even though I walk through the valley of the shadow of death, I will fear no evil, for you are with me" (Psalm 23:4).

God doesn't ask us to go through the dark valleys alone just to promise to meet us on the other side. He assures us that He will go through those valleys with us. And we are never asked to pitch our tent and live in the valleys either. Please be encouraged friend, that the valley you may now be experiencing is just a path to higher ground. My favorite word in all of Psalm 23 is the word "through". God doesn't say that we die in the valley or even get stuck in the valley. "Even though I walk **through** the valley of the shadow of death, I will fear no evil" (v.24). What an encouragement! If you are in a deep dark valley, be assured that you will be able to one-day say like the Psalmist, "He lifted me out of the pit of despair, out of the mud and the mire. He set my feet on solid ground and steadied me as I walked along" (Psalm 40:2).

Even though Lori went home with the Lord, those pearly gates were the ultimate higher ground, and God walked through the whole journey with her.

5. You can ask God "WHY?", but God is under no obligation to respond

> "My thoughts are nothing like your thoughts," says the Lord. "And my ways are far beyond anything you could imagine. For just as the heavens are higher than the earth, so my ways are higher than your ways and my thoughts higher than your thoughts.
>
> Isaiah 55:8-10

Ultimately, God is bigger than what our minds can comprehend and he constantly calls us to trust him through our questions. We are reminded that God is the sovereign one, God is all knowing, God is in charge and he loves us. Instead of asking God the "why" question, try asking God the "what" or "how" question. What is it that you are trying to teach me in this situation? How can I grow to trust you more through this hardship?

The Lord will show you because He *wants* you to grow and learn through adversity.

Job was a man who really struggled with the why question. His three friends were really good friends when they kept silent. Sometimes the best thing you can do for friends who are suffering is to just sit in silence with them. When Job's friends started offering advice, their only conclusion was that Job had grievously sinned and he needed to repent. Finally, Job became worn down and went to the Lord with his questions. In Job chapters 38-41, God addresses Jobs why question. He begins the longest monologue on all of Scripture with these words: "Who is this that questions my wisdom with such ignorant words? Brace yourself like a man, because I have some questions for you, and you must answer them (Job 38:2-3). Basically, God says, "Job, why are you questioning your Creator? You have no idea what you are talking about! Let me ask you some questions". God then answers Job's questions with more questions. God was trying to give Job a proper perspective on His own power and sovereignty. I would encourage you to read those four chapters anytime your circumstances feel overwhelming or hopeless. What is the answer to Job's questions? It's God. *God is the answer.* J.B. Phillips wrote a book called "Your God is Too Small". That's the problem with many of us. We have too small of a view on God and when God is small, our problems are big. The Lord helps Job by enlarging his view of his Creator and by the end of the conversation Job is no longer asking the why question. He simply says,

"I know that you can do anything, and no one can stop you. You asked, 'Who is this that questions my wisdom with such ignorance?' It is I—and I was talking about things I knew nothing about, things far too wonderful for me. You said, 'Listen and I will speak! I have some questions for you, and you must answer them.' I had only heard about you before, but now I have seen you with my own eyes. I take back everything I said, and I sit in dust and ashes to show my repentance." (Job 42:2-6).

That's what happens when our view of God is adjusted so that we can see properly. God gets bigger and our problems become smaller.

6. Let God be in control of our lives.

Lori may have penned one of the main lessons learned through this experience when she wrote to a young friend:

At the start of life we all begin on the summit of a tall mountain. For those who do not accept God's love the top of the mountain is all they experience. They walk in endless, futile circles. Those who accept God's love expand their vision and are able to see His glory down the side of the mountain. Some desire control in their life and choose to descend with grappling hooks and rope. They repel down the side of the mountain trusting in the safeguards they have put in place.

However, they often find themselves tangled and caught in their own rope. Sometimes they find the rope is too short to reach the bottom. The wise Christian realizes to fully experience God's love, grace and provision in life; you must turn from the view down the mountain and fall backward off of the mountain believing God will guide you safely to the bottom. For it is in this freefall that God provides eagle's wings and allows us to soar and explore the life He has given. There is never danger when we trust God because we are ever in the palm of His hand.

God's Word also instructs us. Look here, you who say, "Today or tomorrow we are going to a certain town and will stay there a year. We will do business there and make a profit." How do you know what your life will be like tomorrow? Your life is like the morning fog—it's here a little while, then it's gone. What you ought to say is, "If the Lord wants us to, we will live and do this or that" (James 4:13-15). It's so important for us to live our lives under the rule of God. God is completely sovereign. That means nothing happens in the universe without his knowledge *or* permission. If you are a child of God, then not only does God control your life, He designed it to work in a specific way in a specific order so that you will grow in your faith in Him and bring Him the most glory.

Because my faith was challenged, I have become a different man. And I like it. I have learned to enjoy life more and yet hold it much more loosely. I have learned that there are very few guarantees in this life. "Seventy years are given to us! Some even live to eighty. But even the best years are filled with pain and trouble; soon they disappear, and we fly away. Teach us to realize the brevity of life, so that we may grow in wisdom." (Psalm 90:10,12). It's amazing, but I now no longer worry about things. I lost what was then the most important treasure on this earth, and I have lived to talk about it. Not only that, but my faith is stronger and I no longer battle earthly fears. "So we can say with confidence, 'The Lord is my helper, so I will have no fear. What can mere people do to me?'" (Hebrews 13:6).

7. Life is Hard

"Dear friends, don't be surprised at the fiery trials you are going through, as if something strange were happening to you. Instead, be very glad— for these trials make you partners with Christ in his suffering, so that you will have the wonderful joy of seeing his glory when it is revealed to all the world."

1 Peter 4:12-13

Little did the disciples know at the time but rowing that boat in the midst of a huge storm was just the beginning of the troubles they would face. Life is hard there's no doubt. Because of sin, we have three enemies to our soul: Satan, "the world" and our flesh. Those three opponents wage war against the part of us that seeks to love God with all of our heart. Life is hard because we are at war against the world, the Devil and ourselves. God allows a certain amount of trials in our life with the hopes that we will cling to Him and acquire His assistance to overcome those tribulations.

Charles Spurgeon said that whatever the weight of the trial, equal or surpassing is God's grace and consolation. We had seen that to be true up to this point and we had confidence in His faithfulness. In what do we put our trust? We put our trust in God. We trust him even when we don't understand because He is in control of everything just like He was in control of the waves crashing over the disciples boat.

8. Faith is Trust in God's love, not certainty in God's will

"Trust in the Lord with all your heart;
do not depend on your own understanding.
Seek his will in all you do,
and he will show you which path to take."
(Proverbs 3:5,6)

When it's all said and done, there's a lot more being said than done! But it all comes down to faith. Are we going to trust God and His Word or are we going to allow our circumstances to redefine who God is? According to 1 John 4 verses 8 and 16, God is love and He always acts in love, we cannot allow our trials to alter what the Bible says about the character of God. Because God is love, He always acts in love. If we trust in Him, and not rely on our own understanding or our own interpretation on our circumstances, then Proverbs 3:5 promises us that God will give us the guidance we need so that we are not fumbling in the darkness. But living in faith takes work. The American novelist Mary Flannery O'Connor exclaimed, "Don't expect faith to clear things up for you. It is trust, not certainty."[1]

9. God prioritizes character over comfort

"Consider it pure joy, my brothers, whenever you face trials of many kinds, because you know that the testing of your faith develops perseverance. <u>Perseverance must finish its work</u> so that you may be mature and complete, not lacking anything" (James 1:2-5)

Though our trials are painful and even seem cruel, they are an expression of God's love, not His displeasure. Because God's number one priority is to make us holy, we are going to experience many agonizing trials in this life. These trials should not push us away from the Father's heart, but instead should bring us to our knees in total dependence on God for strength. As we endure the hardships of this life by God's grace, we will find that we will be maturing spiritually, developing among other things patience, peace and perseverance. That's why James tells us to think about our difficulties with joy. Through life's troubles, we are becoming more and more like Christ, and that spiritual maturity has wonderful rewards. It brings with it, peace and joy, and new opportunities to minister to others who go through similar circumstances.

10. God will usually give you more than you can handle.

The goal? To get you to rely on God.

"My health may fail, and my spirit may grow weak, but God remains the strength of my heart;

he is mine forever...
how good it is to be near God!
I have made the Sovereign Lord my shelter."
Psalm 73:26-28

Do not believe it when people tell you that God will not give you more than you can handle. It's just not true. The Lord certainly gave Lori and I more than we could handle even though we did it together. But with each overwhelming circumstance, we found the Lord to be more than enough for our every need. My prayer all along in writing this book has been that you the reader would find comfort in knowing that you are not alone in your trials and that the same God who comforted us will comfort you and with Him in you, there is nothing that the two of you can't handle together. Don't try to do it alone. You were not created to do that. But just like the apostle Paul, you can say with confidence "For I can do everything through Christ, who gives me strength (Philippians 4:13).

Even though we always carry the scars of hurts and losses in our lives, even though we always miss those we have lost, the pain does heal over and life does go on. Dying and suffering are part of our experience on earth because we live in a broken and fallen world. Consider what Jesus said, "I have told you these things, so that in me you may have peace. In this world you will have trouble. But take heart! I have overcome the world." (John 16:33) Because of sin, we have three enemies to our soul: Satan, "the world", and our flesh. These opponents are waging war against us every day. They seek to pull our attention away from loving God with all of our heart. Lori's sickness and death was a profound loss for me and for my children. We could have allowed her death to pull us away from God, but instead we used it as a steppingstone toward God.

After a difficult winter of grief there were hints of spring in the air. The days started getting longer and warmer and before I knew it, there were signs of life everywhere. The changing seasons in the Northeast are a quarterly reminder that life also has its seasons. The winters of our lives can be harsh and hard. Looking around in the winter you have to wonder if anything will ever grow again. What a miracle it is to see the flowers pop out of the ground and leaves sprout from the trees again. It must be a message of hope from God. No matter how hard life can be the springtime of the soul is always right around the corner.

Rachel graduated from high school and went on to post secondary education. Joshua is completing his education and making plans for his own future. I was able to find my way back to routine living and working again. Eventually, I met another beautiful woman who was truly a gift from God. We married and blended our families together in a union that is truly blessed and for which I am truly grateful. My wife Deb and our *three* children have brought me great joy and contentment and remind me daily that the Lord is good.

Life still has its trials. Within a few years of losing Lori my brother-in-law had a massive heart attack and died at the age of 40. Again my family and I were presented with a choice to respond in anger and confusion at God or to trust and have faith in His goodness to us in spite of difficulty.

We continue to press forward and believe that whatever lies ahead is in God's control. He will never leave us or abandon us and no matter what may come His love covers and guides us. We look forward to the day when we can join Lori, along with all the saints and the angels dancing before God's throne.

"And from the throne came a voice that said, 'Praise our God, all his servants, all who fear him, from the least to the greatest.'Then I heard again what sounded like the shout of a vast crowd or the roar of mighty ocean waves or the crash of loud thunder: 'Praise the Lord! For the Lord our God, the Almighty, reigns. Let us be glad and rejoice, and let us give honor to him. For the time has come for the wedding feast of the Lamb, and his bride has prepared herself. She has been given the finest of pure white linen to wear.' For the fine linen represents the good deeds of God's holy people. And the angel said to me, 'Write this: Blessed are those who are invited to the wedding feast of the Lamb.' And he added, 'These are true words that come from God.'"

Revelation 19:5- 9

Bible Study

Chapter 1 Bible study

It has been said, "diamonds are a girls' best friend." Why do women love diamonds so much? Is it that they just love to wear jewelry and are so happy when someone finally gives them something beautiful to wear? The phrase has less to do with the jewelry and more to do with the sentiment behind the jewelry. When I proposed to Lori I offered her a diamond ring as a way of expressing my love. Diamonds are beautiful and valuable and reflect these aspects of love between two people. Diamonds are a good choice for other reasons as well. The journey of a diamond, like the journey of love, is not an easy path. Diamonds start as pure graphite 90 to 100 miles below the earth. The molecular structure of graphite is weak because there aren't many bonds between the molecules. After millions of years of being exposed to temperatures reaching 2,000 degrees Fahrenheit and pressure 50 times greater than that found on the surface of the earth more bonds are formed between the molecules and the structure actually changes and a diamond is finally formed. After it's formation it could take another 1,000 years for diamonds to make it to the earth's surface. Once at the surface someone has to find it, extract it from the ground and eventually send it to the jeweler who then carefully cuts it and creates beautiful jewelry. Most couples reap the benefits of the last step of the diamonds journey without giving any consideration to the long and difficult road taken by the diamond to the jeweler's case. In the same way they do not know the difficulties that await them in marriage. If the two are committed together to withstand the heat and pressure ahead of them their marriage can also become as beautiful and refined as the engagement diamond. The diamond can be a continual reminder of not only love but also the difficulties that lie ahead and the beauty that awaits after withstanding the pressure and heat.

The marriage relationship is designed for so many wonderful reasons. One of those reasons is to reflect God's love for each of us. Just like the diamond and just like marriage our relationship with God will also go through many difficulties. His final objective is to burn away impurities, create strong bonds and reveal the true beauty of his creation, you and me. This requires the intense heat of life, unbearable pressures and an unwavering commitment to make the long journey.

This sounds like a tall order, but God strengthens us and guides us in our journey.

God strengthens us:

Read the first part of 2 Chronicles 16:9, Psalm 89:21, Isaiah 41:10

What message is God giving us in these verses?

How does God accomplish this? Ephesians 3:16

_____

Acts 15:32

_____

Can you recall a time in life when you felt strengthened by someone or something? Write what happened here

_____

_____

God's guidance:

See Philippians 4:4-9

There are several commands given in these verses. Write down all you can identify here:

_____

_____

_____

There are also several results listed. What are they?

_____

_____

What do these verses say about who will guide us?

John 16:13

_____

_____

Isaiah 58:11

_____

_____

Can you recall a time when you received guidance you were sure was from God? Write it here: _____

_____

_____

As you walk the path laid out for you it is encouraging to occasionally recall God's intervention on our behalf or for the sake of others. When you write these events in a journal you can easily recall them. Give some consideration to buying a journal, if you don't already have one, and get into the habit of recording your thoughts, your discoveries and how God moves in your life. When you look back on what you wrote it is easy to see how God strengthens and guides us.

Chapter 2 Bible Study

Throughout the Bible God reveals himself as a holy God who does not abandon us in difficulties. In fact, God knows that we need him before we know that we need him and He often goes out of his way to make his presence known even before tragedy strikes. Lori's sprained ankle was not a tragedy, but the storm clouds were gathering to rain down the true reason for her injury. She didn't know at the time why God was reaching out to her, but in spite of her limited understanding He still reached out to fill her with faith. We can all rest assured that God knows what we need and will reach out to us in many ways even if the road is unclear to us.

Let's consider another woman whose faith was strengthened in difficulty through a visit from an angel.

Read Genesis Chapter 16.

1. How and why was Hagar suffering? _____

_____

_____

This was no fault of Hagar's yet she still found herself in a place of suffering. God sent an angel to Hagar who delivered instructions to her.

2. What are the instructions? _____
_____
_____

And she was to name her son _____
which means _____.

3. After instructing Hagar about what to do she recognizes that God is the God who _____? Write out verse 13 here _____
_____
_____

In Hebrew El Roi.

4. Besides instructions on what to do next God communicated clearly to Hagar through two names, one she gave her son, which means _____
and one she gave to God, which means _____
_____.

When Hagar returned back to Abram she had clear direction and a clear understanding that God is a God who hears and a God who sees her. He did not abandon her to die in the desert, but He provided a way through the desert and led her back to Abram. This was the path God chose for her. These two revelations are truths we also can embrace for our own lives today.

Seldom do we get to see with our very eyes a glimpse of heaven. We believe because of faith that God is in heaven, there are angles singing before God's throne and there is a place prepared for us. The vision Lori had that day was a reassurance to her that her hope of eternal life was not a hollow hope, but rather a hope backed by the power of God revealed to her in a very dramatic way. This glance into heaven was God's way of sending the foundational pilings of her faith deep into the ground so that when the storm grew fierce her faith would remain strong. God often reveals himself to people who are facing trials or need a reassurance of faith. Sometimes He is dramatic in His revelation; sometimes He is the quiet whisper in the wind. God sees our story from beginning to end and provides for us long before we know we even need His provision. God sees us. God knows what's down the road. God has His plan in motion even before we get out of bed and His provision is never too late. Just think of Abraham, Moses, Elijah, Mary, Joseph and the apostle Paul. The personal appearance of an angel of the Lord to these people gave them a great hope and instilled a new measure of faith that would be needed in the days ahead. God's hand was always stretched out to them. He walked close to Abraham and Moses through their difficult journeys and He walks with us too.

It wasn't until much later that I realized what an encouragement that Sunday morning experience was for Lori. It was just one of dozens of ways the Lord let her know she was loved. God gave Lori a great gift of supernatural sight and it became a source of life to her soul.

This source of life is available to all of us. God has promised us that we will never walk alone. God is a holy

God and yet He reaches out to us and is ever present with us. This is the wonder of the gospel, that we as sinners are separated from God because God's holiness cannot tolerate sin. Through Christ we are once again united with God. Listen to the way the apostle Paul puts it:

> "But God showed his great love for us by sending Christ to die for us while we were still sinners. And since we have been made right in God's sight by the blood of Christ, he will certainly save us from God's condemnation. For since our friendship with God was restored by the death of his Son while we were still his enemies, we will certainly be saved through the life of his Son. So now we can rejoice in our wonderful new relationship with God because our Lord Jesus Christ has made us friends of God" (Romans 5:8- 11)

Once we belong to Him, He never abandons us. His comforting presence is forever with us and can manifest itself in some fascinating ways. Consider this verse:

> But now, O Jacob, listen to the Lord who created you. O Israel, the one who formed you says, "Do not be afraid, for I have ransomed you. I have called you by name; you are mine. When you go through deep waters, I will be with you. When you go through rivers of difficulty, you will not drown. When you walk through the fire of oppression, you will not be burned up; the flames will not consume you. For I am the Lord, your God..." (Isaiah 43:1-3).

I believe that "vision," communicated to Lori that our Father in Heaven was close, very close, to her. All she needed to do was look up for help, strength and grace.

"I lift up my eyes to the hills — where does my help come from? My help comes from the LORD, the Maker of heaven and earth (Psalm 121:1-2)

Although He sometimes allows painful trials in our life, He wants us to know that He absolutely *will* be there for us to lean on for strength, courage, and even joy (Nehemiah 8:10). The way God communicates His presence in our lives will vary from person to person, but be rest assured, God will never leave us or make us face our trials alone. He will let you know that He is alive and working in your life.

For more encouragement about how God is with you through your darkest times read Psalm 139:7-12.

Chapter 3 Bible Study

This chapter opens with a lot of unanswered questions. Everyone was trying to make sense of this physical affliction. There seemed to be no reason for it. The doctors were running tests as Lori's condition grew worse each day. Anger, doubt and unbelief throw a party under these conditions. There is a choice to make at this point of the journey. Will you give in to these negative emotions toward God or will you push deeper into prayer and into God's Word to wait patiently for his answers?

Pain, like pleasure, has the potential to choke out God's Word in our life, block us from hearing God's answers and destroy our faith. That is not what God has in mind for us. Think back to the parable of the sower (Matthew 13:1-23). Jesus tells us that one of the ways the seed (God's Word) is choked out is by the rocky soil, which represents trials or persecution. At first the seed/God's Word is received with joy and it springs up very quickly. But it doesn't have any root so that when the hard times come, that plant is choked out.

We need to give God's Word every chance to grow in our lives and that means the soil in our lives needs to be fertile. When we hear or read the Bible, it has the power to penetrate the deepest parts of our being, changing the way we view life's circumstances. The Bible offers help, hope, and healing, and when we read it daily, it builds our faith.

2 Timothy 3:16-17tells us that "all Scripture is inspired by God and is useful to teach us what is true and to make us realize what is wrong in our lives. It corrects us when we are wrong and teaches us to do what is right. God uses it to prepare and equip his people to do every good work."

We have already seen how God reaches out to us in a variety of ways and we've already learned that God sees our situation and hears our prayers. He sees the bigger picture that we don't see. Let's take a look at someone else who did not have all the answers and who also had a decision to make.

Read I Samuel 1:1-20

Answer these questions as you think about your own response to God in your difficulties.

1. V. 5 why did Elkanah give a double portion of the meat to Hannah?

a. _____

b. _____

The LORD has closed her womb. The LORD allowed this hardship to come upon Hannah for a reason. The hardships He allows to come to us are always for a reason.

2. V. 6 How does the bible characterize Peninnah and what did she do to Hannah?

_____

_____

v. 7 How often did this go on? _____

v. 8 Her husband loved her. Did he understand her situation? _____

3. v. 9 - v. 15 What was Eli's initial response to Hannah?

_____

It's clear that Hannah had to review her situation and make a choice. She was unable to have children. The Lord brought this on her himself, she had someone in her life who constantly taunted her in order to irritate her. Even the priests in the temple accused her of being drunk and her own husband didn't understand her grief. She was all alone in her pain and suffering. Who could have blamed her if she had chosen to doubt God and be angry with him?

4. What did Hannah do in spite of all her pain and unanswered questions? _____

_____

5. What can we learn from Hannah's example?

_____

_____

The Bible is God's very Word to us. Hannah believed that God is good and would speak to her and He did. He speaks to each of us today as well and always answers our prayer even if it's not what we want to hear. We must approach the Bible with a teachable spirit. Try praying King David's prayer: "Open my eyes to see the wonderful truths in your instructions."(Psalm119:18)

Chapter 4 Bible Study

We read and studied in Chapter 1 that God is with us every step of our lives. He sees us, He hears us and He walks with us. No matter how much we know about God and believe in his Word the moment of devastating news is an inconsolable moment. Fear, confusion and anger are all normal responses. At that point you do your best to make it home safely and then turn to pillars of strength in your life. Family and close friends are an immediate source of comfort and strength and it's a good idea to include even a Pastor into the immediate aftermath of bad news. Picking up a Bible at this time is a good choice but may not be everyone's first choice. Even for the most scholarly of Bible students focusing on relevant Scriptures verses may prove to be a challenge. It is a good time to lean on the strength of trusted people in your life.

The disciples also faced death in a boat one day. They were fearful and angry and had to learn an important lesson about trusting God in the midst of the storms of life.

Luke 8:22-25 tells the story of how Jesus calmed the storm.

1. The disciples were fine in the boat until a sudden storm came upon them. What "storm" has suddenly come upon you or a family member? _____

_____

2. The waves grew bigger, the disciples looked around at their situation and saw large waves crashing over their lifeboat. What "large waves" do you see crashing over you?

_____

3. The wind grew stronger and they tried as hard as possible to steer that boat against the storm.
The disciples heard the wind roar around their boat. What does the "wind" sound like to you? _____

_____

4. There was no steering the boat, though, because the storm was too big, the waves were too high and the wind was too strong. They had no control over their circumstances. They were terrified at what might happen. Think of your situation. What is your deepest fear? What is your deepest hurt? What are you angry about? Share those thoughts with God. _____

_____

If you are wrestling with frustration and anger (I am finding out that most of my so-called "frustration" is just suppressed anger wrapped in a façade of gentleness), I want to encourage you to take it to the cross. It is only there at the feet of Jesus that we can lay down our feelings of injustice and even sometimes the desire for vengeance (see Romans 12:19-21). I find it very hard to stay angry with someone for whom I pray. Jesus challenges us to do exactly that "Bless those who curse you. Pray for those who hurt you."(Luke 6:28) Christianity is not for the faint-hearted or weak-minded. The way of the Cross is a life of self-denial, putting others before yourself all in the name of loving God with all that you are and loving your neighbor as yourself (be it a godly or godless individual) (Matthew 22:27-40).

It is possible to trust God in the midst of confusion and anger. Trust is simply putting confidence in God. Trust is directing your actions, prayers and responses according to God's Word rather than according to your emotions. People put trust in various comforts or assurances, but if these do not have a foundation in God they will surely crumble. "Some trust in chariots and some in horses, but we trust in the name of the LORD our God." (Psalm 20:7) The disciples for example, found themselves in a difficult situation. They trusted in their strength to row and steer the boat against the storm. When they realized that their own strength was crumbling and they had no control over the wild sea they called out to Jesus and discovered that He was trustworthy because He had power and control. This was a big lesson for the disciples and a big lesson for us today. The question we face each day is, "Who is going to be in charge of my life?" Some might say, "I'll be in charge of my own life. I'm smart and strong and educated. I think I can handle my own life." Some might think of a counselor or a pastor. Some may think of an overbearing boss. Still others may think of a disease or disability that seems to dictate every move of the day. None of these has the same authority as God in our life. God is Lord over everyone and everything, and if we acknowledge that He is the one guiding us and worthy of our trust we can save ourselves the disappointment that will surely come upon discovering all the others crumbled. We have the benefit of God's Word to instruct us in advance that He is trustworthy and He has not abandoned us in difficult circumstances. He walks very close to all who call on his name.

They called for Jesus, who was asleep in the stern and Mark 4:38 says, "The disciples woke him and said to him, "Teacher, don't you care if we drown?" Jesus was able to sleep because He had no fear and was sure of the outcome of the situation. What appeared unknown and scary for the disciples was very clear to God. He woke up and rebuked the waves, calmed the storm and asked the disciples "Why are you so afraid? Do you still have no faith?"

Take a minute in your own heart and say a prayer that puts you and your loved ones under the knowing strength of God. Place yourself in the "boat" of your life and look at the "waves" (whatever is crashing in on you today) and listen to the "wind" (whatever bad news you hear). Then think about the fact that Jesus knows exactly what is going to happen. He has all of your lives in the palm of his hand. He walks very close to each and every one of you. He sees every passing minute and hears every desperate sigh. No matter what trouble comes your way God is there to strengthen, comfort and be with you. You are not left alone in your circumstances.

Take some time to write about the day you received your bad news. As you write think about Jesus who stands to command the sea and the wind and know He can also command and order your life as well.

_____

_____

_____

_____

_____

_____

_____

_____

Chapter 5 Bible Study

John 11:1-43 records the story of Lazarus. After reading the passage answer the questions.

1. Do you get the sense that Jesus was a friend to Mary, Martha and Lazarus? What makes you think so?

_____

_____

2. What was Jesus' response to the news that Lazarus was sick?

_____

3. How does Jesus' response strike you? _____

_____

4. What does it mean to bring God "glory"? When you look in the dictionary you might find terms like "renown", "fame", "prestige", "honor", "acclaim", "recognition", "worship", "adoration". The essence of bringing glory to God is making him known on earth. Our experiences can be used to reveal his prestige, honor, fame, acclaim etc. This was the purpose for Lazarus's sickness.

Notice Jesus did not say, "Lazarus will not die" he said, "This sickness will not end in death". The burning question remains.

Why would Jesus allow his friends, who must have been like family to him, go through this bitter pain?

_____

_____

What do you think this says about our purpose on earth? _____

_____

It might have been difficult for Mary and Martha to have faith in Jesus after their brother died. It is difficult for us to have faith, sometimes, as we look at our own circumstances. Faith is trust in God's love, not certainty in God's will. When we assume to know God's will, we leave the door open for disappointment, as we will inevitably misinterpret it. When we TRUST in God's LOVE for us, we know that no matter what happens He is guiding our circumstances exactly as He has decided.

Lori and I did not know God's will for this journey with ALS. We certainly had our preferences, but we trusted in His unfailing love for us, no matter what happened. When you exercise your faith during suffering and hardships, you are in essence telling God, "Lord, I don't know why this is happening, when it's going to stop, or what the end result will be, but I know that you love me, and all of this will be redeemed by you and used for my good and your glory." Trusting in God's love is confidence in the character of God, not the will of God. Most often, God asks us to trust him when we don't know where He's leading. Sometimes Jesus just says, "Follow me"; the rest of it is a faith walk.

"Trust in the Lord with all your heart; do not depend on your own understanding. Seek his will in all you do, and he will show you which path to take." (Proverbs 3:5).

5. When Jesus found out that Lazarus was sick He did not rush right out to heal him. He was not that far away and could have gotten to Bethany quickly. How do you think the family felt when they sent word for Jesus to come and He did not? _____

_____

Lazarus was passing literally in the shadow of death and Jesus did nothing about it. What could have been some of the responses from Mary and Martha toward Jesus? _____

_____

6. Verses 17 - 27 Record Martha's response to Jesus. What was her response and how is it like or unlike your own response to him in the Valley of the Shadow of Death? _____

_____
_____
_____
_____
_____

7. Verses 28 - 36 Record Mary's response to Jesus. What do you observe about her interaction with him?

_____

_____

_____

_____

8. What do you observe about his interaction with her and how it was different than his interaction with Martha? _____

_____

_____

_____

We may not understand why Jesus doesn't come immediately when we call to him from the darkness of our soul. It may look like He is taking his time for no apparent reason. Mary and Martha had no idea why Jesus didn't come to Lazarus immediately. If that were me, I might have gotten a little angry. I might have even taken the "thanks a lot" attitude with God. "You healed everyone else, but you couldn't take the time to come to those of us who are like family to you?" There is a plan though. We rarely get the benefit of seeing the entire plan all at once, but we can be sure God does have one. Sometimes in sickness and difficulty the plan is to bring glory to God. It may seem harsh that God would allow someone to get sick so that He can be revealed on earth. The question looms, "Couldn't He find another way? Why let people get sick? Why let people die? There is no other way for God to reveal himself to the world?" God chooses to use the hands and the feet of the people He created. One of our purposes in being here is to bring glory to God. This is a hard concept to accept when someone gets sick or loses their job or has a bad accident. If we realize that we came from God, we belong to Him, and He has redeemed us from death then we can grasp the idea easier that we are here to bring Him glory. As we submit to His authority as a merciful Creator then we can take the attitude of Paul who wrote to the Romans, "For from him and through Him and to Him are all things. To Him be the glory forever! Amen." (Romans 11:36) God is the source, the sustainer and the goal of all things. Everything that happens in our life ultimately comes down to the glory of God. "So whether you eat or drink, or whatever you do, do it all for the glory of God." (1 Corinthians 10:31)

9. How can we have such confidence when everything seems to be going bad? Romans 8:28 _____

_____

_____

_____

This is not a band-aid verse we try to apply to someone's wound that is in a desperate circumstance. Rather, this is an attitude we acquire after a long journey of struggling to understand why God allows some of us to pass through the deepest darkest valley of death. The key to a peaceful walk through the dark valley is to believe that God has a plan, He shares in our pain and in the end everything works for the good of those who love him.

10. Verses 38 - 43 What happens at the end of this story? _____

The plan God chose for Lazarus was healing and resurrection. He created that plan for with a purpose. He may not plan the same for others, but we can be confident that He does have a unique plan for each of us. We remember both Lazarus and Jesus were raised from the dead and we too will one day be called forth from the grave. Go ahead and boldly pray for resurrection. It may not come when you would want, but it will come for each and every one of us who have the hope of eternity written on our hearts with the blood of Jesus.

Chapter 6 Bible Study

We were created for community plain and simple. We need each other. As I look back at those difficult months, I just don't know how I would have made it emotionally, spiritually, or financially if it were not for the body of Christ.

God has equipped each person with gifts and abilities in order to play a unique and important role God's plan.

Read 1 Corinthians 12

v. 4 There are different kinds of _____ _____   _____ _____ but the same _____ the same _____ the same _____,

v. 7 Tells us why each manifestation of the Spirit is give:
_____

v. 14 - 31 makes an analogy between how the body works as one unit and how God's people also work together to carry out his plan. Can you think of your-self and other people in your life and notice how God is moving everyone together for one purpose? Explain.

_____

_____

_____

_____

_____

What are we instructed to do according to according to 1 Timothy 6:18-19? When we do this what is the result?

_____

_____

_____

_____

For some of us it is very difficult to receive help from others. It may seem too dependent or weak. The bible commands us to help others according to the gifts we have received. Sometimes we are the helper and some-times the receiver. No one is exempt from needing help. So, if you need help don't be ashamed to accept it from those who are gifted to provide what you may need at the time. When you are able then you do what you can to help someone else. In this way everyone can be taken care of.

In my experience, most churches respond well to a short-term crisis. I watched for many years as volun-teers prepared meals, provided babysitting, shuttled children, gave financially or visited someone in the hospital. The Lord has given the church all it needs to fully function as a community of grace and love. We are not mere "volunteers". We are all ministers called to serve one another.

In the case of long term needs helping someone for an extended period of time can be a challenge. It will require structure and direction from the leaders of the church so that those who are able to help can do so in an efficient and appropriate manner. How can this be done?

Stephen Ministry (www.stephenministries.org) equips lay caregivers (called Stephen Ministers) to provide one-to-one Christian care to the bereaved, hospitalized, terminally ill, separated, divorced, unemployed, relocated, and others facing a crisis or life challenge. They provide all the training necessary in order to launch the ministry in your church, no matter what size your congregation may be. At the very least, there needs to be a core group of people who can take a good hard look at the needs of the individual or family and assess what the church can do for them.

Chapter 7 Bible study

We had been holding on to the hope of a healing for months but Lori's condition just continued to deteriorate. At some point the reality of an unanswered prayer can take it's toll on your faith. Some people pray and God answers them exactly as requested. Other people pray and the answer is, "no". When the answer is no it really makes a person question God's motives. "Could a loving God really allow this to happen?", "He could change all of this with one word, why doesn't He do something?" "Doesn't He care about me or my family?" These are legitimate questions with no easy answers. Let's take a look at a few examples of others who were sick and expected God to intervene.

Read John 9:1-12 about the man who was born blind
1. What question did the disciples ask him?

_____

_____

2. What was Jesus' response to them? _____

_____

_____

3. Is it fair that the man had to endure the suffering imposed on him all those years by being blind?

_____

_____

4. If God allowed him to suffer for a reason how can this change our outlook on affliction? _____

_____

We tend to think of God strictly in terms of his loving character. There are so many aspects of God's character to explore. What do you think of a God who allows you to be afflicted for his own purposes? _____

_____

_____

_____

5. Read Mark 14:32- 41

Jesus also cried out to his Father in suffering. What did He ask his father to do? _____

_____

6. What was his Father's response? _____

_____

Jesus knew that his suffering and death were for a higher purpose. It is difficult to accept the fact that the Father would send his very own Son to die. He had the authority and the power to take away the suffering, but He didn't. You can be sure the Father suffered along with him knowing there was no other way. The world we live in is laden with sin. The effects of sin have touched every thing that ever lived on this earth. Even Jesus bore the weight of sin on the cross. Sickness, disease and suffering don't originate in God they originate in evil. God in his sovereignty chooses very carefully what He allows to touch the lives of his children. He allows only those things that will ultimately serve a higher purpose in our lives and in his kingdom.

Is this to say we shouldn't pray for healing? Not at all! We should pray for healing and believe that God can heal. There are numerous examples in the Bible of how God healed people. Even at the hour of Jesus' death many of the tombs broke open and the bodies of holy men came back to life. God is in the business of giving life. When our prayers aren't answered the way we want it's an occasion to exercise deeper faith in God and believe that He has a perfect plan. We can pray that our own hearts are refined because it's in the crucible of trials that the dross of misplaced affections are exposed and burned away. For this reason we can embrace suffering as a means of becoming more like Christ. We can pray that something good comes from the sickness. We can pray that God would be revealed through this hardship. This is the attitude Paul had when he said " Remember Jesus Christ, raised from the dead, descended from David. This is my gospel for which I am suffering even to the point of being chained like a criminal. But God's Word is not chained." (2Timothy 2:8-9) Paul understood that his suffering was for a reason and even though his body was in chains God's Word is never chained. The kind of suffering we endure today may be different than Paul, but the outcome can still be the same. God allows us all to suffer; it is our attitude and willingness to turn it around for God's glory that makes the difference in the outcome. In this way, whether physical healing occurs or not God still works a miracle. The miracle is that his glory is revealed to everyone on earth through the willing hearts of his servants.

God was revealed very clearly as Lori held on to her faith in the midst of her trial, as people around us served selflessly, as the love in my own heart grew and provide me the strength to take care of her and as a peaceful man wept at the feet of one of God's beloved. Through all of this, God showed that He desires to be emotionally and practically involved with our suffering. He is ready to work a miracle. We need to be ready to accept the miracle He sends.

Chapter 8 Bible study

The months around the holidays are usually filled with thoughts of family and love. They can be a joyous time of celebration with expressions of thanks, and exchanges of gifts. The holiday season for us that year was laden with expressions of love. Lori expressed her love to everyone with words, we exchanged gifts, we spent time celebrating and we thoroughly enjoyed our time together. Even a complete stranger, Joni, was able to communicate God's love for us through a timely letter. These exchanges of sincere care and gratitude made great family photos and terrific memories. We should remember that love is much more than a warm feeling on a special day. Love is a very powerful force in the lives of all people. Everyone who is the recipient of a sincere act of love is changed. We are commanded by God to love one another. Why is this so important? It's important because love draws us closer to God, sustains our hearts and minds, and lifts us up even as disease and suffering may be pulling us down. Consider these commands we find in God's Word.

Be devoted to one another in brotherly love. Honor one another above yourselves. Romans 12:10

Let no debt remain outstanding, except the continuing debt to love one another, for he who loves his fellowman has fulfilled the law. Romans 13:8

You, my brothers, were called to be free. But do not use your freedom to indulge the sinful nature; rather, serve one another in love. Galatians 5:13

Now that you have purified yourselves by obeying the truth so that you have sincere love for your brothers, love one another deeply, from the heart. 1 Peter 1:22

Love has the power to set people free, to breathe life into tired souls and to embrace a broken heart. Love has the power to comfort the sick, encourage the downhearted and embrace the lost.

Read Matthew 22:34-40

1. What did Jesus say is the greatest commandment?

_____

_____

2. And the second greatest commandment? _____

_____

_____

Lori spent the time she had left making sure that her family and friends knew she loved them and they did the same for her. Sometimes communicating such love is not easy because harsh words or actions may have gotten in the way over the years. In the end, the most important part of life is love. Here are a few difficult questions to consider:

* Given my current circumstances am I doing what I can to show those around me that I love them?
* Is there someone who needs to hear an expression of my love that hasn't heard it in a while?
* How can I express my love for God in my situation?
* How is God expressing His love to me my situation?

I want to encourage you to seize every opportunity to express your love as much as possible. Once someone is gone then it's too late to say it or show it. Don't let a single chance slip by to let people around you know that you love them and care about them. As you do this you can be sure that you are fulfilling God's commands. Maybe James Taylor said it best in his song:

Just shower the people you love with love
Show them the way that you feel
Things are gonna work out fine if you only will
Shower the people you love with love
Show them the way you feel
Things are gonna be much better if you only will [2]

Showering others with love while under the burden of pain and suffering may seem like an impossible request on top of everything else God tells us to do. How can we find the energy to think of others while in the midst of our own struggle? How can God require so much of us? Doesn't it seem like sometimes God requires more of us than we could ever possibly accomplish? The fact of the matter is God will usually give you more than you can handle. In our own hearts and minds we are sincere in wanting to accomplish everything on our own strength. We want to do what pleases God. We fail to realize that at the end of our best effort we still will fall short of the tall order God has laid before us. This is not to say we shouldn't work our hardest, but maybe we can realize along the way that God will empower us to do what He has required. This is why He says,

> " Come to me, all you who are weary and burdened, and I will give you rest. Take my yoke upon you and learn from me, for I am gentle and humble in heart, and you will find rest for your souls. For my yoke is easy and my burden is light." (Matthew 11:28-30)

The yoke is easy because He carries the burden of suffering with us, He provides the strength to accomplish all that is required of us for each day, He fills us to overflowing with his love and we share that with others. The key to success is to rely on God. Consider this verse: "My health may fail, and my spirit may grow weak, but God remains the strength of my heart; He is mine forever... how good it is to be near God! I have made the Sovereign Lord my shelter..." (Psalm 73:26-28) When our health fails or our spirit grows weak, we can believe that God is our strength and shelter. In Him we find all the power we need to love each other, to worship in joy, to serve and to accomplish the tasks He has for us no matter how big or small.

Chapter 9 Bible Study

The darkness of winter provided the perfect cover for the kids and me to grieve. We spent a lot of time together as a family and allowed that time to bring whatever healing it could offer. I'm not sure that the pain of losing someone you love ever really goes away. I am sure it doesn't disrupt life forever. Hope offers a respite from the pain. One of the greatest aspects of Christianity is hope. We have hope of salvation and believe that Lori is in heaven. We have hope in the resurrection from the dead for all who believe. We have hope that in heaven every tear is wiped away and there is no more sickness or pain. We have hope that one day we will see those we love again. Take courage from these words:

> "Brothers, we do not want you to be ignorant about those who fall asleep, or to grieve like the rest of men, who have no hope. We believe that Jesus died and rose again and so we believe that God will bring with Jesus those who have fallen asleep in him. According to the Lord's own word, we tell you that we who are still alive, who are left

till the coming of the Lord, will certainly not pre-cede those who have fallen asleep. For the Lord himself will come down from heaven, with a loud command, with the voice of the archangel and with the trumpet call of God, and the dead in Christ will rise first. After that, we who are still alive and are left will be caught up together with them in the clouds to meet the Lord in the air. And so we will be with the Lord forever. Therefore encourage each other with these words." (1 Thessalonians 4:13- 18 NIV)

What promises does God make in these verses? Which verse offers you the most comfort or hope? Why?

_____

_____

_____

We take comfort in the fact that the Lord was so inti-mately involved in Lori's life and death. There is no indication that God abandons us at the time of death, but rather is ever present with us.

Read Psalm 16:15 and record what it says here:

_____

God sees each person and notices each death. We can also be sure that it has been appointed to each man to die once (see Hebrews 9:27) and after that there's hope of life. Once a person passes through death, it loses its power. The person throws off the binding chains of death and lives in heaven free from the fear of ever dying again.

We can also be sure that God is there to grieve and to comfort in our time of loss. As we have seen Jesus himself grieved at the loss of his dear friend Lazarus. As we read in Psalm 62:8 God desires for us to pour out our hearts to him. Record those words here as a reminder.

_____

What does God promise us in Isaiah 44:3?

_____

_____

_____

We can see that God sandwiches death in between two experiences of life. He walks with each person through the dark valley, out the other side and straight into eternal life. He also provides comfort and peace to those who are left on earth. Death may seem like a dark abyss, but in reality there is life permeating every step of the process. God is and always will be a life giver.

Chapter 10 Bible Study

The hope of eternal life covered our family along every step of our journey. This hope is not a hollow, powerless hope, but rather a hope backed up by the Word of God. It is a hope full of heaven's authority and it is trustworthy. This hope comes to us through the love of Jesus who gave himself so we could understand the Good News. He gives each of us a choice to believe the good news or not. What is this good news? Paul said it best when addressing the people of Athens. His words are recorded in Acts 17:24-34

> "He is the God who made the world and everything in it. Since he is Lord of heaven and earth, he doesn't live in man-made temples, and human hands can't serve his needs—for he has no needs. He himself gives life and breath to everything, and he satisfies every need. From one man he created all the nations throughout the whole earth. He decided beforehand when they should rise and fall, and he determined their boundaries.

"His purpose was for the nations to seek after God and perhaps feel their way toward him and find him—though he is not far from any one of us. For in him we live and move and exist. As some of your own poets have said, 'We are his offspring.' And since this is true, we shouldn't think of God as an idol designed by craftsmen from gold or silver or stone.

"God overlooked people's ignorance about these things in earlier times, but now he commands everyone everywhere to repent of their sins and turn to him. For he has set a day for judging the world with justice by the man he has appointed, and he proved to everyone who this is by raising him from the dead."

When they heard Paul speak about the resurrection of the dead, some laughed in contempt, but others said, "We want to hear more about this later." That ended Paul's discussion with them, but some joined him and became believers"

1. Who is the Lord of heaven and earth? _____
_____

2. V. 25 says that God gives all men _____
and _____ and _____

3. V. 26 says God determined the _____
and the exact _____ where
each person would _____

4. V. 27 Why did God determine these things?

_____

_____

Verse 27 also says that God is not _____ from each of us.

5. V. 28 In him we _____ and _____ and _____.

6. V. 30 God commands each person to _____.

7. V 32 says that upon hearing the message some people _____ but some people _____

Just as the people of Athens had a choice each of us is presented with a choice as well. Are we going to sneer like some of the people from Athens or are we going to be like Dionysius and Damaris who believed that God is near and is calling us to repent? Even Jesus commanded people to repent because the kingdom of God is near.

> "When Jesus heard that John had been put in prison, he returned to Galilee. Leaving Nazareth, he went and lived in Capernaum, which was by the lake in the area of Zebulun and Naphtali— to fulfill what was said through the prophet Isaiah:
> "Land of Zebulun and land of Naphtali,
> the way to the sea, along the Jordan,
> Galilee of the Gentiles—
> the people living in darkness
> have seen a great light;

on those living in the land of the shadow of
death
a light has dawned."
From that time on Jesus began to preach, 'Repent,
for the kingdom of heaven is near. '"

Matthew 4:12-17

God's message is clear to us and this is the Good News, the Gospel. Jesus has made a way for us to repent of sin and make peace with God. He desires so much for us to come to him that He chooses very carefully the place in which we live and the time in which we live so as to give us the best opportunity to repent and embrace him. He is always close by each of us waiting for the time when we decide to place our trust in his Lordship over our lives. He is the power behind the hope of eternal life. It is God who will supply all your needs both for this life and the suffering and hardship it brings, and for the next life in heaven.

If you have not put your trust and faith in Jesus this would be a great time to take that step of faith. He has chosen the time and place for you to live in hope that you will come to him. Maybe this book at this time is meant for you. If you would like to place your trust in Christ take a minute now and say this prayer to God. A sincere and willing heart is all that it takes.

God, I believe that you have designed my life very carefully and you are calling me to repent and receive your kingdom. I acknowledge that there has been sin in my life. I accept that Jesus, dying on the cross for me, has received the penalty for my sin and because of his obedience I can be free to be one of your own. I renounce sin and commit myself to be obedient to your Word. I accept what Christ did for me and commit myself to your Lordship. Thank you for sending me the Holy Spirit, who will remind me of everything Jesus taught, is a guide and comfort to me for the rest of my life. Amen

Endnotes

Chapter 10
(1) Mary Flannery O'Connor, The Habit of Being (New York: Farrar, Strauss and Giroux, 1979), 354.

Chapter 8 Bible Study-
(2) "SHOWER THE PEOPLE" Written by: James Taylor Performed by: James Taylor 1976
Appears on: "Shower the People" B-side: "I Can Dream of You" 45RPM 1976; In the Pocket-1976, Greatest Hits-1976 Classic Songs-1990, Live in Rio-1991; James Taylor: Best Live-1994; '70s Folk Rock-1995*; Chicken Soup for the Soul: The Collection-1998*; Live at the Beacon Theater (CD & Video)-1998; The Best of James Taylor-2003; One Man Band-2007; et al.

Breinigsville, PA USA
23 June 2010
240487BV00001B/2/P